Understanding Pneumoviruses: The Potential of PVM as a Research Model

Anton

First Printing, 2024

Table of contents

1. Introduction 1

1.1 The pneumonia virus of mice 2

1.2 Genomic organization 2
1.2.1 The PVM particle 2
1.2.2 PVM genome organization 3

1.3 The PVM proteins 4
1.3.1 The small hydrophobic protein, SH 5
1.3.2 The G glycoprotein 6

1.4 Transcription, replication and pathogenesis of the pneumoviruses 9
1.4.1 Transcription 9
1.4.2 Replication and pathogenesis 10

1.5 Reverse genetics for the pneumoviruses 11

1.6 PVM strains 12

1.7 Propagation of PVM 14

1.8 PVM as a surrogate model of RSV 15

1.9 Translational regulation of protein synthesis by the upstream open reading frame 16

1.10 Aim and objectives of the book 16

2. Materials and Methods 17
2.1 Viruses, Mice and Materials 17
2.1.1 Mice 17
2.1.2 Viruses 17
2.1.3 Cells 17
2.1.4 Media for cell culture 18
2.1.5 Plasmids 18
2.1.6 Competent cell and media 18
2.1.7 DNA and RNA modifying enzymes 19
2.1.8 Primers 19
2.1.9 Restriction enzymes 20
2.1.10 Purified antibodies and antisera 20
2.1.11 Commercial kits 20
2.1.12 Laboratory instruments 21
2.1.13 Chemicals 22
2.1.14 Plastics wares and other consumables 23
2.1.15 Solutions and buffers 24
2.1.16 Computer software 26

2.2 Methods 27
2.2.1 Cells 27
2.2.2 Virus propagation 27
2.2.3 Virus quantification by plaque assay 28
2.2.4 Replication kinetics in tissue culture 28

2.2.5 Amplification of a PVM J3666 fragment spanning M to F genes (J3666-MSHGF) ... 28
2.2.6 Molecular cloning of J3666-MSHGF ... 30
2.2.7 Generation of pPVM-G_{J3666}65A and pPVM-G_{J3666}65U plasmids ... 32
2.2.8 Isolation of rPVM-G_{J3666}65U and rPVM-G_{J3666}65A from plasmids ... 33
2.2.9 Western blot analysis of protein ... 34
2.2.10 Quantitative polymerase chain reaction (RT-qPCR) ... 36
2.2.11 Animal experiment ... 37
2.2.12 Statistical analysis ... 37

3. Results ... 38

3.1 PVM J3666 represents two distinct populations ... 38

3.2 Contribution of the PVM-G gene organisation to replication and virulence ... 42
3.2.1 Generation of recombinant PVM containing the G_{J3666}65A and G_{J3666}65U ... 42
3.2.2 The G gene organization affected the expression level of the G protein ... 45
3.2.3 Effects of the J3666-G gene variants on multicycle replication kinetics in tissue culture ... 46
3.2.4 The composition of the G gene affects the virulence of PVM in BALB/c mice ... 48

3.3 The G gene determines the replication phenotype of biological PVM strains ... 50
3.3.1 Selection of individual PVM-J3666 populations by sequential passaging in tissue culture 50
3.3.2 The level of G protein synthesis differs between biological PVM isolates ... 51
3.3.3 The biological PVM isolates exhibit different replication kinetics in tissue culture ... 53

3.4 **Recombinant PVMs encoding a N-terminus truncated G protein or lacking the G gene are attenuated in macrophage-like cells due to the level of their G glycoprotein expression** ... 56
3.4.1 The level of G protein expression correlated with incorporation into virus particles ... 56
3.4.2 The replication efficiency of PVM in RAW 264.7 cells correlated with G protein levels ... 58
3.4.3 Attenuation of rPVM-ΔG-GFP and rPVM-Gt is specific for macrophages ... 61

4. Discussion ... 64
4.1 The quasispecies of PVM J3666 represents two distinct populations ... 64
4.2 Influence of the 5' untranslated region on G protein expression ... 66
4.3 The effects of G expression levels on replication in cultured cells ... 69
4.4 The effect of G expression level on virulence and replication in vivo ... 71

5. Conclusion and perspective ... 73

6. References ... 74

1. Introduction

The family *Paramyxoviridae* is subdivided into the subfamilies *Pneumovirinae* and *Paramyxovirinae*. These subfamilies differ in size, genome organization, nucleocapsid content, and arrangement of the glycoproteins on mature virions. The *Pneumovirinae* is further divided into the genera *Pneumovirus* and *Metapneumovirus*. The members of genus *Pneumovirus* contain two additional non-structural genes and the attachment protein gene, G, is not adjacent to the polymerase gene as for those in genus *Metapneumovirus* (King et al., 2012).

The type species of the genus *Pneumovirus* is the human respiratory syncytial virus (RSV), a major cause of acute lower respiratory tract infections in infants and children worldwide and more recently identified as an important pathogen in immunocompromised adults (Walsh, 2011). Unfortunately, RSV has no suitable laboratory animal model that mimics the natural infection, as a result many aspects of the viral life cycle have not been studied in the host-pathogen context (Bem et al., 2011). The pneumonia virus of mice (PVM) is a natural pathogen of mice that shares many features with RSV such as genomic arrangement and functionally homologous genes. Therefore, PVM has been proposed to be a suitable surrogate model to study the pathogenicity and immunological properties of RSV in a natural host-pathogen context (as reviewed by Easton et al., 2006; Dyer et al., 2012), however, there are gaps in our understanding of the virus.

One of the main antigenic proteins of the RSV is the G protein, a type-II glycoprotein that has been suggested to be the main attachment protein. It is also used for classification of strains and subgroups due to its high sequence divergence (Anderson et al., 1985; Mufson et al., 1985; Johnson et al., 1987). This protein has been implicated in immune evasion and modulation but the main function is yet to be determined (reviewed by Collins, 2011). The RSV G gene is structurally similar to the PVM G gene but contains a shorter open reading frame (Easton et al., 2006).

Three strains of PVM, J3666, 15 and Y, have been described in the literature. The complete nucleotide sequences of the genome of PVM J3666 and the two substrains of PVM 15 as well as the partial sequence of PVM Y have been determined. Phylogenetic analysis of the sequences indicated that these PVM strains contain different G gene arrangement (Dyer et al., 2012). Furthermore, the specific polymorphism responsible for the variation in pathogenesis between the virulent and avirulent substrains of PVM 15 was mapped to the sequence composition of their G genes (Krempl et al., 2007).

Therefore, this project was designed to understand the effects of the polymorphisms in the structure of the PVM G on gene expression, replication, and virulence as a step to further our understanding of function of the G glycoprotein in the pneumoviruses.

1.1 The pneumonia virus of mice

PVM was isolated from healthy Swiss mice when nasopharyngeal washings from patients with non-influenza diseases were serially passaged in mouse lungs. It was later understood that the pneumotropic virus was not from the passaged human suspension but a latent pathogen of the mouse lungs that gained virulence during the serial passaging in lungs of mice (Horsfall and Hahn, 1939; Horsfall and Hahn, 1940). Today, PVM is now recognized as one of the several pathogens of laboratory rodent colonies, where it causes apparent infections in rodents, especially mice and rats. The mechanism of the virus spread in these colonies are yet to be resolved as infected mice are mostly unable to transmit the virus to uninfected mice placed in the same litter (Horsfall and Hahn, 1940; Horsfall and Curnen, 1946; Zenner and Regnault, 2000). This is unlike RSV infections that are easily transmittable through close contact.

Natural PVM infections have been reported in athymic mice used as sentinel mice (Richter et al., 1988; Weir et al., 1988; Miyata et al., 1995) as well as in other rodents such as hamster and rats (Miyata et al., 1995); and non-rodents such as dogs, rabbits, cats and hedge dog (Miyata et al., 1993; Renshaw et al., 2010; Glineur et al., 2014; Madarame et al., 2014). Also, several studies have reported PVM-specific antibodies in sera from different sources, including humans (Horsfall and Hahn, 1940; Horsfall and Curnen, 1946; Pringle and Eglin, 1986; Miyata et al., 1993; Zenner and Regnault, 2000). However, a more detailed approach showed that PVM is probably not a human pathogen due to the high replication restriction of recombinant PVM in the lungs of African green monkeys and rhesus macaques, and absence of seroconversion in these animals. The study also found that the human sera do not react specifically with any PVM protein (Brock et al., 2012).

1.2 Genomic organization

1.2.1 The PVM particle

PVM is a single-stranded, non-segmented, enveloped, and pleomorphic RNA virus that replicates primarily in the cytoplasm of infected cells like RSV. Unlike RSV, PVM has been suggested to cause agglutination of the red blood cells, which appears to be a special feature of its G glycoprotein (Ling and Pringle, 1989). Nonetheless, PVM and RSV share similar genomic arrangement of their genes, replication pattern, reduced stability at elevated temperature and high susceptibility to ether treatment (Easton et al., 2006; Dyer et al., 2012).

Compans and colleagues using virus purified from BHK-21 cells showed that PVM virions occur as spheres or filaments and sometimes as pleomorphic particles within an envelope that is host-derived. The envelope are covered with virus-specific glycoprotein spikes as shown in Figure 1 (Compans et al., 1967). Later, Berthiaume and colleagues (Berthiaume et al., 1974) confirmed these observations using virus particles purified from Vero cells and further showed that the filamentous form was the most prevalent. The spikes on PVM virions were more tightly packed with only a distance of 6 nm as against

10 nm between spikes found on RSV virions that were mostly spherical. However, the size, arrangement, and morphological appearance of the nucleocapsids of RSV and PVM within the envelope were very comparable (Berthiaume et al., 1974).

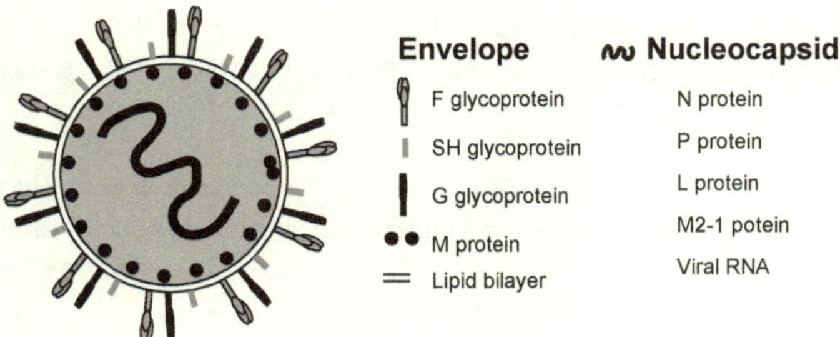

Figure 1: Graphic representation of idealized PVM particle.
The homo-oligomers of the viral glycoprotein spikes, the nucleocapsid, the lipid bilayer, and the matrix protein are shown. The diagram is not drawn to scale nor does it depict the exact spatial arrangement. The image was adapted from the chapter: Respiratory syncytial virus and metapneumovirus in volume one of the 5th edition of Field's virology edited by Knipe and Howley (Collins and Crowe, 2006).

1.2.2 PVM genome organization

PVM has the typical linear genome of non-segmented negative-stranded RNA viruses, with a size ranging from 14,885 to 14,887 base pairs. The genes are arranged in the genome as shown in Figure 2 (Krempl et al., 2005; Thorpe and Easton, 2005). Many of PVM proteins are assumed to be analogous to those of RSV (Chambers et al., 1990).

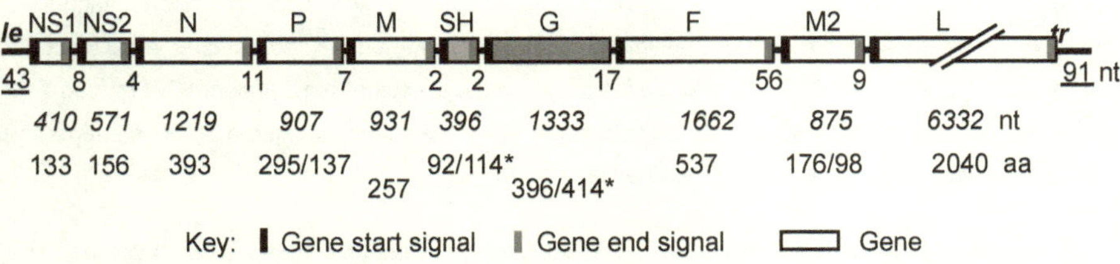

Figure 2: Linear representation of the genome of pneumonia virus of mice.
Genes are shown as rectangles, with the shaded bars at each end representing the gene-start and gene-end transcription signals. The length of the leader (le) and trailer (tr) regions in nucleotides (nt) is shown at ends of the genome with the underlined numbers. The length (in nt) of the intergenic sequences between the genes is shown below them with the first row of numbers; the length of each gene (in nt) and the respective number of amino acids (aa) are shown below in the second and third rows, respectively. The P and M2 genes contain two open reading frames (ORF) within their genes and two possible ORF length described for the SH and G genes are shown and indicated by asterick. The image was adapted from the chapter respiratory syncytial virus and metapneumovirus in the volume one of the 5th edition of Field's virology edited by Knipe and Howley (Collins and Crowe, 2006).

At the 3' and 5' ends of the genomic RNA are the leader and trailer regions, respectively, which are not transcribed into mRNA. The leader sequence encodes signals for replication and transcription of the viral RNA whereas the trailer signal is only involved in replication. The 10 genes between the leader and trailer regions are spaced by a non-conserved intergenic sequences (IGS) ranging from 2 to 56 nt (Chambers et al., 1991; Krempl et al., 2005). In a RSV minigenome system, IGS were found not to play a role in regulation of gene expression (Kuo et al., 1996a) and by analogy, PVM IGS are also thought not to affect gene expression.

There are gene-start (GS) and gene-end (GE) signals at the 3' and 5' ends of each gene to guide the virus-encoded polymerase to initiate and terminate transcription, respectively. In addition, the U tract sequence in the gene end signal ensures the polyadenation of the nascent mRNA (Collins, 2011). The arrangement of the genes is believed to reflect the amount of each gene product required, since transcription of virus genes occurs in a gradient-like manner, with genes at the 3' end of the genome being more transcribed than those at the 5' end. The linear map of the PVM genome shown in Figure 2 like those of RSV includes the two non-structural proteins: NS1 and NS2 that are rarely found in purified particles. However, certain differences have been reported between the genome of RSV and PVM. PVM P gene unlike its counterpart in RSV contains at least two major open reading frames, P-ORF1 and P-ORF 2 (Barr et al., 1994). In addition, the M2 and L genes of PVM do not overlap as in the human or bovine RSV (Krempl et al., 2005; Thorpe and Easton, 2005).

1.3 The PVM proteins

The PVM NS1 and NS2 are the most abundant transcribed mRNAs due to their proximity to the 3' end of the genome (Chambers et al., 1990). These proteins have been implicated in inhibition of interferon-I and–III responses (Buchholz et al., 2009; Heinze et al., 2011). In addition to interferon antagonism, RSV NS1 protein was associated with inhibition of transcription and RNA replication in a minigenome system (Atreya et al., 1998). The replication-dependent attenuation of recombinant RSV lacking NS2 gene in both upper and lower respiratory tracts of chimpanzees also suggested a possible role for the NS2 protein in virus replication (Whitehead et al., 1999).

The morphological appearance of the nucleocapsid complex of pneumoviruses differs from the other members of the *Paramyxoviridae* (Berthiaume et al., 1974). The PVM nucleocapsid complex consists of the genomic RNA, nucleoprotein N, phosphoprotein P, large protein L and M2-1 protein. The M2-1 protein is not found in other genera within the subfamily *Paramyxovirinae* and as such is not present within their nucleocapsid complex (reviewed in Easton et al., 2006). The RNA-dependent RNA polymerase (RdRp) consisting of the L and P is required for transcription and replication of the virus genome. In RSV, the viral RNA is always encapsidated by the N protein and bound to the RdRp via its interaction with the P protein (as reviewed by Collins, 2011). Like in RSV, this interaction between PVM P and N proteins appeared to involve both the carboxyl and the amino termini of the PVM P protein (Easton et al., 2006). By analogy to M2-1 and M2-2 proteins of RSV, the PVM M2-1 protein is required for generation of full-length transcripts of all genes and generation of viable virus while the shift between replication and transcription of the genomic RNA is controlled by the M2-2 protein (Ahmadian et al., 2005). During replication, the RSV nucleocapsid complex is found within the cytoplasmic inclusion, from where the complex interacts with the matrix protein via the M2-1 protein. Once bound to the M, the nucleocapsid complex is transported to the cell surface for packaging into the newly formed host-derived envelope containing the glycoproteins (Ghildyal et al., 2006).

The PVM M protein shares about 42% homology to its counterpart in RSV and less to those found in the *Metapneumovirus* (Easton and Chambers, 1997). Nevertheless, hydropathy profiles and function of the M genes of several genera from different virus families of the non-segmented negative-strand RNA virus seemed to be comparable (Latiff et al., 2004). The M protein of other paramyxoviruses appears to be the major determinant of virion morphology (Curran and Kolakofsky, 1999). The RSV M protein is usually found lining the inner wall of the virus envelope as shown in Figure 1 (Marty et al., 2004) and is required for formation of RSV particle (Teng and Collins, 1998; Mitra et al., 2012). RSV M protein is thought to transverse into the nucleus to shut-off host protein synthesis during the early phase of RSV infection (Ghildyal et al., 2003; Ghildyal et al., 2009). During RSV particle assembly, the M protein is assumed to inactivate the transcriptase activity in preparation for assembly (reviewed by Ghildyal et al., 2006) and subsequently brings the nucleocapsid complex within the cytoplasmic inclusion into the newly formed envelope (Ghildyal et al., 2002; Li et al., 2008). Furthermore, the RSV M protein has been shown to interact with the viral glycoproteins that are located within the host-derived envelope (Henderson et al., 2002; Ghildyal et al., 2005a; Shaikh et al., 2012).

PVM expresses three glycoproteins on its surface: the fusion protein F, the attachment protein G, and the small hydrophobic protein SH. These glycoproteins are responsible for many of the important functions of the viruses such as receptor binding, immune evasion and generation of neutralizing antibodies (McLellan et al., 2013). The F glycoprotein directs the fusion of the virus particles with the host cell membrane, allowing virus entry into the host in a pH independent manner. The F protein is a type-I single-pass integral membrane protein that is cleaved into two subunits: F_1 and F_2, by trans-Golgi endoproteases from the initial precursor, F_0, that is the primary translational product (Ling and Pringle, 1989b; Chambers et al., 1992). The PVM F protein alone is sufficient to support the entry, replication, and release of viable viruses in the absence of the G protein (Krempl et al., 2007) as described for other pneumoviruses (Karger et al., 2001; Teng et al., 2001; Biacchesi et al., 2004).

1.3.1 The small hydrophobic protein, SH

The SH gene has the smallest open reading frame (ORF) that codes for a type-II integral membrane glycoprotein. The PVM SH protein ORF is larger than the RSV SH ORF and shorter than the human metapneumovirus (hMPV) ORF. PVM SH protein contains more potential N-linked glycosylation sites (4 sites) compared to the RSV SH protein (2 sites) and hMPV SH protein (1 site). Also, the amino- and carboxy-termini of the PVM SH protein are hydrophobic compared to RSV SH protein with only one hydrophobic domain at the amino-terminus (Easton and Chambers, 1997).

The composition of SH gene is divergent between strains of PVM but the molecular size of the SH protein are somewhat similar. The SH mRNA of PVM strains 15 and Y codes for a polypeptide of 92 amino acids whereas the J3666 SH mRNA can code for a polypeptide of either 92 or 114 amino acids (Thorpe and Easton, 2005; Genbank acc. No. JQ899033.1). Although, there is no report on the direct function of the PVM SH in tissue culture or in vivo, it is believed that it is functionally similar to the homologous proteins found in other pneumoviruses (Easton et al., 2006). The RSV SH protein plays no role in virus binding to the host cells (Techaarpornkul et al., 2001; Schlender et al., 2003) but appeared to inhibit TNF-α response in tissue culture (Fuentes et al., 2007). In addition, the SH protein was reported to function as viroporin (Collins and Mottet, 1993; Triantafilou et al., 2013) and to affect plaque formation in a cell line-dependent manner (Bukreyev et al., 1997) as well as inhibition of syncytia formation in the absence of the G protein (Bukreyev et al., 1997; Techaarpornkul et al., 2001). The RSV SH protein interacts directly with the G glycoprotein but not with the F glycoprotein (Feldman et al., 2001; Low et al., 2008) while the human metapneumovirus SH and G proteins were reported to work together to prevent uptake of the virus by dendritic cells *in vitro* (Le Nouen et al., 2014).

Recombinant RSV deficient for the SH gene was successfully recovered but it was attenuated in the lower respiratory tract of chimpanzees (Whitehead et al., 1999) and upper respiratory tract of mice (Bukreyev et al., 1997). Furthermore, the deletion of the SH gene in the avian metapneumovirus severely affected virus production and immunogenicity (Ling et al., 2008). All these observations indicated that the SH protein is important for maintaining virulence in animals even though it is indispensable for replication in tissue culture.

1.3.2 The G glycoprotein

The PVM-G is a mucin-like, type-II transmembrane glycoprotein (Ling and Pringle, 1989b) analogous to RSV-G (Wertz et al., 1985). The RSV G protein has N-linked and O-linked glycosylation sites, accounting for 60% of the molecular weight observed on SDS-PAGE gels and for antigenic variation and immune evasion (Anderson et al., 1985; Mufson et al., 1985; Lambert, 1988; Garcia-Barreno et al., 1989; Waris, 1991). This glycosylation affected the overall molecular weight in a cell-specific manner (Garcia-Beato et al., 1996; Kwilas et al., 2009). By analogy to the RSV-G protein, the PVM-G glycoprotein was regarded as the main attachment protein (Ling and Pringle, 1989b). The main receptor for PVM-G protein is yet to be determined but heparin had been suggested as the possible receptor for both the human and bovine RSV-G proteins (Levine et al., 1987; Feldman et al., 1999; Karger et al., 2001). In contrast to the RSV-G protein, PVM-G proteins can also act as viral hemagglutinins (Compans et al., 1967; Ling and Pringle, 1989b).

The PVM 15 G is synthesised in two glycosylated forms identified as G1 (M_r ~ 76.4 kDa) and G2 (M_r ~ 62 kDa), the G1 form is thought to be the precursor for the G2 variant (Ling and Pringle, 1989b). Both forms are present in virus particle in contrast to the RSV G with one membrane-anchored form inserted in the virion and a second secreted form released by infected cells into the culture medium (Hendricks et al., 1987; Hendricks et al., 1988). The secreted RSV G protein is translated from the second start codon located within the signal/anchor sequence and then undergoes a post-translational cleavage by proteolysis that remove the amino-terminus (Hendricks et al., 1988). Analysis of the antigenic properties of the secreted and membrane bound RSV-G proteins using panels of monoclonal antibodies found no difference between both forms of RSV-G glycoproteins (Escribano-Romero et al., 2004). The secreted form of RSV was assumed to be responsible for evasion of early immune responses in mice (Bukreyev et al., 2008), modulation of immune responses (Johnson et al., 1998; Arnold et al., 2004; Schwarze, 2004) and prevention of antibody-mediated inhibition of RSV replication *in vivo* (Bukreyev et al., 2008; Bukreyev et al., 2012). The deletion of the secreted G protein in recombinant RSV was also reported to attenuate the virus in mice (Maher et al., 2004).

The G protein of PVM strains identified so far contains between 363 and 414 amino acids due to variations in the length of their potential cytoplasmic domain (Randhawa et al., 1995; Krempl et al., 2005). In contrast, the difference in the length of RSV G protein containing between 282 and 321 amino acids is due to polymorphisms in the ectodomain region (Wertz et al., 1985; Trento et al., 2003; Eshaghi et al., 2012). The G mRNA of PVM 15/ATCC codes for a protein containing a cytoplasmic domain of 35 amino acids while the cytoplasmic domain is truncated in the avirulent variant of PVM 15/ATCC, designated PVM 15/Warwick, due to insertion of an extra nucleotide (Randhawa et al., 1995; Krempl and Collins, 2004). The extra nucleotide caused a frameshift mutation that moved the translation initiation from the first AUG encompassing the predicted cytoplasmic domain to the downstream AUG closer to the signal/anchor sequence (Randhawa et al., 1995). Randhawa and colleagues (Randhawa et al., 1995) also reported a PVM J3666-G mRNA containing an upstream ORF (uORF) coding for a polypeptide of 12 amino acids before the main G ORF that would be translated into a G protein comprising of a 35 amino acids cytoplasmic tail as shown for PVM 15/ATCC. This PVM J3666-G mRNA is similar to RSV-G mRNA. RSV-G mRNA contains an uORF of 15 amino acids that slightly overlaps the main G ORF (Wertz et al., 1985). The uORF before the RSV-G ORF somewhat reduces the amount of the translatable product from the main G ORF but otherwise does not affect its functions in cell culture (Teng et al., 2001). A second variant of PVM J3666-G gene was described in which the uORF and the downstream ORF were fused to single ORF by a point mutation that ablated the stop codon of the uORF, to potentially encode a G protein that contains an extended cytoplasmic domain of 53 amino acids (Krempl and Collins, 2004). Interestingly, this form of G gene is also found in the only PVM strain, strain Y, isolated from diseased mice (Weir et al., 1988; Genbank acc. No. JQ899033.1) and those of the newly isolated canine pneumoviruses, CnPnV, recovered from diseased dog suffering from canine infectious respiratory disease (Renshaw et al., 2010; Glineur et al., 2013; Decaro et al., 2014).

Currently there is little information on the direct role of cytoplasmic tail of the PVM-G protein. A recombinant PVM from which the part of the G gene coding for the cytoplasmic domain was deleted suggested that it is not important for replication in mice or *in vitro*. However, the replication-independent attenuation of the virus led the authors to conclude that the cytoplasmic domain is likely a virulence factor required for intracellular signalling (Krempl et al., 2007). Studies on the role of the cytoplasmic tail of other type-II viral glycoproteins: RSV G (Ghildyal et al., 2005b); hemagglutinin-neuraminidase of parainfluenza virus type 3 and Newcastle disease virus (Spriggs and Collins, 1990; Wilson et al., 1990); influenza virus A neuraminidase (Garcia-Sastre and Palese, 1995; Zhang et al., 2000) and several other glycoproteins have shown that the cytoplasmic tail contributed to intracellular trafficking and the interaction of fully processed protein with other viral proteins. The absence of the cytoplasmic tail in influenza virus hemagglutinin glycoproteins affected replication in tissue culture and mice (Garcia-Sastre and Palese, 1995). Some of these studies also highlighted the importance of the length of the cytoplasmic tail in its overall function (Spriggs and Collins, 1990; Wilson et al., 1990).

Generally, there is little conservation between the RSV-G and PVM-G (Figure 3) at nucleotide or amino acids level (Thorpe and Easton, 2005) and their specific antibodies do not cross-react (Brock et al., 2012). The PVM-G protein appears not to contain either the central conserved domain or the CXC3 motif found between the two mucin-like regions of RSV-G protein (as reviewed by Collins and Graham, 2008). Also, the secreted form of PVM-G protein was not detectable in BHK-21 cells infected with recombinant PVM expressing the full-length G protein or the truncated G protein without the putative cytoplasmic domain (Krempl et al., 2007). However, both proteins contain high amount of serine, threonine, and proline residues (Wertz et al., 1985; Randhawa et al., 1995). The predicted secondary structure of the PVM-G protein, its location within the virus genome and replication studies in tissue culture and lungs of infected mice suggested that it should be functionally similar to RSV-G protein (Ling and Pringle, 1989a; Ling and Pringle, 1989b; Krempl et al., 2007).

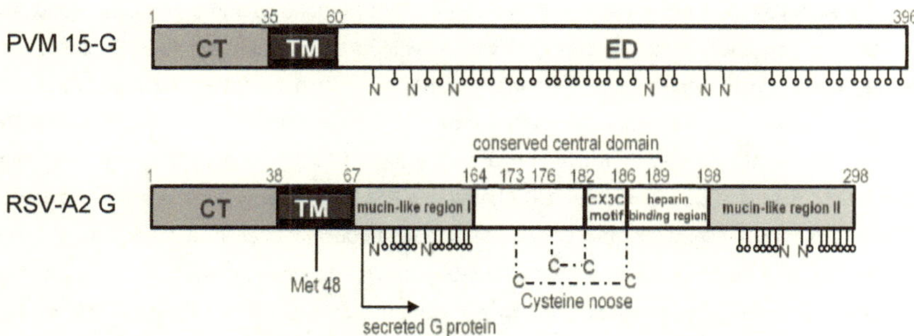

Figure 3: Comparison of the structural features of PVM and RSV G proteins.
Schematic of the RSV-G and PVM-G showing the different parts of the proteins. The cytoplasmic domain, CT; transmembrane portion, TM; the carboxy-terminus, ED and the corresponding length in each G protein are shown. The possible N- and O-glycosylation sites predicted with the GlycoEP (Chauhan et al., 2013) are indicated with N and the small open circles, respectively. The translation initiation site (MET 48) and the N-terminus of the proteolytically cleaved translation product of the MET 48, that is, the secreted G protein are shown. The positions of other known features for the RSV-G protein are also indicated. Of note, the heparin-binding domain is located between amino acids 184 and 198. The figures are adopted from (Krempl et al., 2005; Melendi et al., 2011; McLellan et al., 2013)

RSV-G is required for adequate incorporation of the SH protein into the released virus particle (Batonick and Wertz, 2011); enhancement of fusion activity of the F protein (Techaarpornkul et al., 2001; Techaarpornkul et al., 2002; Schlender et al., 2003) and generation of protective immune response in human (Karron et al., 1997). A study on the direct effect of the PVM-G protein on replication and virulence in mice indicated that the G protein is dispensable in tissue culture but essential in mice as described for RSV and other pneumoviruses (Teng et al., 2001; Schmidt et al., 2002; Biacchesi et al., 2004; Biacchesi et al., 2005; Krempl et al., 2007; Widjojoatmodjo et al., 2010). The PVM glycoprotein G contains CD4 T cell and CD8 T cell epitopes (Claassen et al., 2007; Walsh et al., 2013). Claassen et al., 2007 also reported that the CD4 T cell epitope within the PVM-G gene acts in tandem with the CD8 T cell epitope present within the PVM-P protein to induce protective immunity. Furthermore, the conserved domains and the secreted form of the RSV G glycoprotein that are yet to be identified in PVM-G have been implicated in modulation of immune responses during RSV infection such as recruitment of lymphocytes and leukocytes, determination of type of the T-helper cells to be recruited, inhibition of innate immunity and immune evasion (Melero et al., 1997; Collins and Graham, 2008). The hMPV-G protein was reported to inhibit interferon-type-I and -III induction (Bao et al., 2008; Bao et al., 2013; Banos-Lara Mdel et al., 2015). Similarly, in concert with the SH protein, the hMPV-G was shown to prevent the virus uptake in monocyte-derived dendritic cells leading to poor stimulation of CD4 T cells (Le Nouen et al., 2014).

1.4 Transcription, replication and pathogenesis of the pneumoviruses

1.4.1 Transcription

Of all *Pneumoviruses*, transcription is best described for the type-specie RSV. Transcription of the virus genes starts from the leader region at the 3' end and progresses towards the 5' end in a gradient manner due to the sequential start-stop-restart mechanism of the polymerase (Dickens et al., 1984). Each gene contains a gene-start (GS) and gene-end (GE) signal that allows the polymerase to properly initiate and terminate transcription, respectively (Kuo et al., 1996b; Kuo et al., 1997). The transcription of RSV genes appears to be independent of replication as certain mutations that affect transcription does not affect replication indicating that these two connected processes are probably independent of each other (Fearns et al., 1997; Fearns et al., 2000; Fearns et al., 2002; Cartee et al., 2003; Tran et al., 2004).

The RSV GS sequences are well-conserved and contain signals for transcription initiation (Kuo et al., 1997) while those of RSV GE signal sequences are semi-conserved and contain signal for transcription termination (Kuo et al., 1997; Moudy et al., 2003). The polymorphisms of the RSV GE sequence affect termination efficiency of the polymerase, causing production of dicistronic and multicistronic mRNAs. This is because the polymerase can only initiate the transcription of a new gene after successful recognition of the GE signal of the preceding gene (Kuo et al., 1997; Cartee et al., 2003; Moudy et al., 2003; Tran et al., 2004). Based on the efficiency at which the preceding GE sequences signal the termination of transcription, Hardy and colleagues (Hardy et al., 1999) classified the junctions between the RSV genes into three groups: high termination efficiency (SH/G), moderate termination efficiency (N/P, P/M, M/SH, SH/G, and G/F) and poor termination efficiency (NS1/NS2, NS2/N, M2/L, and L/trailer). Using recombinant RSV mutations within the GE signals were shown to regulate only the transcription of the immediate downstream gene but not the overall mRNA gradient (Tran et al., 2004) in line with findings from RSV biological isolates (Moudy et al., 2003). The author also reported that increasing or decreasing the termination efficiency did not affect replication *in vitro* or *in vivo* (Tran et al., 2004).

Another possible regulatory factor is the intergenic sequence (IGS) between the genes, which length appears not to affect the transcription of a downstream gene in dicistronic plasmids (Kuo et al., 1996a). Though, certain deletions and mutations in biological isolates were reported to affect transcription of downstream genes (Moudy et al., 2004).

The sequences of the GS signals in PVM are also relatively conserved whereas those of the GE signals are semi-conserved (Chambers et al., 1991; Krempl et al., 2005). By analogy to RSV, these signals are assumed to serve similar functions in PVM. However, analyses of the composition of the GS and GE signals of RSV, AMPV and PVM indicated that these viruses might have preferential nucleotide usage at these signals (Kuo et al., 1996b; Edworthy and Easton, 2005; Dibben and Easton, 2007). For example, nucleotide position 9 of PVM GS signals was very tolerant to any type of mutation while same position in RSV and APV were intolerant to any kind of mutation.

1.4.2 Replication and pathogenesis

PVM replication occurs primarily in the cytoplasm of the infected cell (Harter and Choppin, 1967), where the negative-stranded genome is replicated by the virus-encoded RNA-dependent RNA polymerase (RdRp). Little is known on how the PVM RdRp replicates the genome but it is assumed that the replication pattern of PVM would follow similar mechanism described for RSV. The RSV RdRp enters the genome at the leader region and then progresses towards the trailer region to produce the antigenomic RNA that is tightly encapsidated with N protein and subsequently replicated to produce the genomic RNA (reviewed in Collins, 2011).

PVM replicates in discrete cycles that takes about 18 – 20 hours in both nucleated and enucleated cells and does not lead to pronounced cytopathic effects as described for RSV (Berthiaume et al., 1974; Cash et al., 1979). In interferon-competent cell lines such as RAW 264.7 cells, PVM infection leads to induction of inflammatory cytokines including tumour necrosis factor-α, interferon beta response, macrophage inflammatory protein Iα and β, and macrophage inflammatory peptide-2 allowing ex-vivo studies of important aspect of PVM pathogenesis (Dyer et al., 2012). In mouse lungs, PVM replicates in the epithelium and one cycle was calculated to take around 24 - 30 hours to produce a 16-fold increase in virus titre (Ginsberg and Horsfall, 1951). However, using *in situ* hybridization assay, PVM N RNAs were first detected within the lung alveolar space at about 48 hours postinfection (Cook et al., 1998). PVM reaches its replication peak between day 5 and 8 postinfection depending on the mouse strain and the strain and volume of PVM used for infection (Cook et al., 1998; Frey et al., 2008; Watkiss et al., 2013). The increase in titre between cycles was estimated to be relatively constant regardless of the volume of inoculum used (Ginsberg and Horsfall, 1951; Horsfall and Ginsberg, 1951) but the inoculum size determined the time required to reach the peak of infection as well as its severity (Horsfall and Ginsberg, 1951; Cook et al., 1998; Krempl and Collins, 2004; Krempl et al., 2007; Watkiss et al., 2013).

PVM replication in mouse lungs is accompanied by weight loss that is a good marker to monitor disease progression. The degree of weight loss correlates with disease severity, which is a function of the extent of pneumonia and bronchiolitis developed in the lungs of infected mice as a sequelae of the degree of virus replication (Horsfall and Ginsberg, 1951). The degree of weight loss was more pronounced during virus clearance than during virus amplification or at peak of virus infection (Frey et al., 2008) while pneumonia was estimated to increase in severity at around 4.7-fold per day (Horsfall and Ginsberg, 1951). However, when PVM strain 15/Warwick (Domachowske et al., 2002) or recombinant virus expressing G glycoprotein without the putative cytoplasmic tail (Krempl et al., 2007) was used to infect BALB/c mice, high replication in mouse lungs did not induce disease, indicating that the G glycoprotein may also contribute to pathology in a replication independent manner.

1.5 Reverse genetics for the pneumoviruses

Two types of reverse genetic system have been described for the *Pneumoviruses*. One system permits the recovery of infectious virus particles from cloned cDNA transfected into suitable cells while the other involves the use of the minireplicon comparable to truncated genome to analyse the contribution of different portions of the virus genome on the replication cycle (Hoenen et al., 2011; Pfaller et al., 2015; Su et al., 2015). Both systems involve the reconstitution of active ribonucleoprotein (RNP) complex, which is the minimum infectious unit of the pneumovirus from individual RNA generated from the cloned cDNA and trans-added support plasmids expressing viral proteins required for generation of viable virus (Conzelmann, 2013).

The minireplicon system also referred to as the minigenome can either be monocistronic or dicistronic. The minigenome was used as a predecessor of the full-length infectious clone to decipher the *cis*- and *trans*-acting factors required for the encapsidation of the virus particle, replication and transcription of virus RNA and assembly of the minimum replication units required to generate viable virus particles (Collins et al., 1993; Teng and Collins, 1998; Collins et al., 1999; Fearns and Collins, 1999; Fearns et al., 2000; Peeples and Collins, 2000; Fearns et al., 2002; Dibben and Easton, 2007; Dibben et al., 2008). The components of a standard minigenome are: the promoter and terminator sequences of T7 RNA polymerase (T7) to control expression of the cloned cDNA; antisense sequence of the hepatitis delta virus (HDV) ribozyme to ensure precise excision of the cDNA from the T7; antisense cDNA of the leader and trailer regions of the genome; the 5'- and 3'- UTRs of the gene(s) of interest. The open reading frame between the UTRs of the gene of interest is typically replaced with a reporter gene such as chloramphenicol acetyl transferase or luciferase to monitor the level of gene expression. The use of antisense DNA prevents the direct transcription of the minireplicon into messenger RNA by the RNA polymerase. Since the minireplicon cannot drives its own replication and transcription, viral proteins (N, P, L and M2-1 proteins) required for these processes are supplied in *trans* by coinfection with helper virus or more recently by plasmid-encoded viral proteins under T7, which is nowadays supplied by transfected stable cell lines transiently expressing it. Once the minigenome is transfected into appropriate cells, the T7 ensures its transcription into negative-sense RNA that will be encapsidated by the *trans*-added N protein and then by L and P protein to form the active ribonucleoprotein complex required to initiate transcription and replication.

For the generation of a full-length PVM infectious particle, the complete antigenomic cDNA of PVM is placed immediately downstream of a T7 promoter sequence, followed by the hepatitis delta virus ribozyme sequence and then by T7 terminator sequence. This construct is then inserted into a plasmid that can be transfected into BHK-21 cells constitutively expressing T7, alongside the minimum replication unit (N, P, L and M2-1 proteins) supplied *in trans* as described for the minireplicon (Krempl et al., 2007). Once transfected, the T7 transcribe the cDNA into genomic RNA that will be artificially encapsidated by the *trans*-added N protein. The encapsidated RNA can then be recognized by the RNA-dependent RNA polymerase complex to initiate the viral replication cycle. The high fidelity of the T7 polymerase limits the production of quasispecies. *In vitro* DNA sequencing analysis can then be used to monitor the composition of the recombinant virus.

These systems permit the specific analysis of virus genes in a natural background, including the detailed analysis of point mutations on the overall fitness of a virus and introduction of artificial mutations within the biological strains to generate recombinant viruses with desired properties and known history (reviewed in Taniguchi and Komoto, 2012; Stobart and Moore, 2014).

1.6 PVM strains

Horsfall and Hahn reported the isolation of 11 PVM isolates from Swiss mice in their first paper where they described the identification of a virus capable of causing pneumonia in mice. Six of the eleven isolates were described to be immunological identical based on sera cross-reactivity. Although, many of the isolates named numerically (2, 7, 15, 16, 17, 25, 27, 28) were studied in their second paper, they favoured isolate 15 for reasons they did not mentioned other than that the isolate appeared to have varying virulence in mice from different breeders (Horsfall and Hahn, 1940). The isolate was renamed PVM strain 15 and was the only isolate deposited with the American Type Culture Collection (ATCC). Thereafter, PVM 15 was used to establish the replication cycle of PVM in mice (Ginsberg and Horsfall, 1951; Horsfall and Ginsberg, 1951), the genomic arrangement, and expression pattern of the virus proteins in infected cells (Compans et al., 1967; Berthiaume et al., 1974; Pringle and Parry, 1980). The techniques for propagation and production of PVM in tissue culture (Harter and Choppin, 1967) and virus quantification by plaque assay on BHK-21 cells (Shimonaski and Came, 1970) were also developed based on this strain. Another research group reported that possible propagation of PVM 15 in BS-C-1 cells (Cash et al., 1977). However, plaque purification of a clone of the PVM 15 and/or the continuous maintenance of the clone in the BS-C-1 cells led to generation of an attenuated variant now designated, PVM 15/Warwick (Cash et al., 1979; Randhawa et al., 1995). PVM 15/Warwick expresses a G protein without the putative cytoplasmic tail due to insertion of an additional uridine residue that caused a frameshift mutation moving the AUG of the first ORF out of frame from the rest of the G ORF, thus preventing the expression of the cytoplasmic domain (Randhawa et al., 1995).

In 1995, a second strain of PVM, PVM J3666, was described (Randhawa et al., 1995). PVM J3666 was reported to have originated from the same laboratory where the original PVM 15 was first identified (Cook et al., 1998). PVM J3666 was subsequently suggested to be more pathogenic than PVM

15/ATCC, although no direct evidence was provided (Ellis et al., 2007). Of note, the name PVM J3666 differs from the nomenclature used by Horsfall and Hahn (Horsfall and Hahn, 1940) and no information is available on its isolation history in any scientific literature. Nonetheless, PVM J3666 shares all features with strain 15 and sequencing of its complete genome revealed high nucleotide identity (99.7%) and amino acid homology with PVM 15/Warwick (Thorpe and Easton, 2005). However, PVM 15/Warwick and PVM J3666 were shown to induce different immune responses and pathology in mice (Domachowske et al., 2002). Another distinct strain of PVM was isolated from athymic mice during a PVM outbreak in 1988 (Weir et al., 1988). The isolate was described to be similar to PVM 15 based on immunological staining and cross-reactivity with anti-PVM-polyclonal antibody, electron micrographs, and other biochemical studies. The strain was later designated as PVM strain Y and its partial sequence was deposited in GenBank under the accession number JQ899033.1. The high sequence homology between the available partial sequence of this strain and the corresponding portion in PVM 15 confirmed the reported similarities. Recently, a new canine pneumovirus, CnPnV, was isolated from dogs suffering from canine infectious respiratory disease. The analysis of the different CnPnV isolates revealed it close relatedness to PVM at the nucleotide and amino acids levels (Renshaw et al., 2010; Renshaw et al., 2011; Glineur et al., 2013; Mitchell et al., 2013; Decaro et al., 2014). Furthermore, CnPnV isolates replicated efficiently in laboratory mice providing evidence for widespread of PVM-related viruses in other animals (Percopo et al., 2011; Glineur et al., 2013).

Full genomic sequences for PVM J3666 (AY743909.1), PVM 15/ATCC (AY729016.1), the attenuated PVM 15/Warwick (AY743910.1) and partial genome sequence of PVM Y (JQ899033.1) are available in GenBank. There are several nucleotide differences between strains 15, Y and J3666, but the most important differences appeared to be located within the G gene and involve the length and composition of the predicted cytoplasmic tail of the G proteins as shown in Figure 4 (Krempl et al., 2005; Thorpe and Easton, 2005).

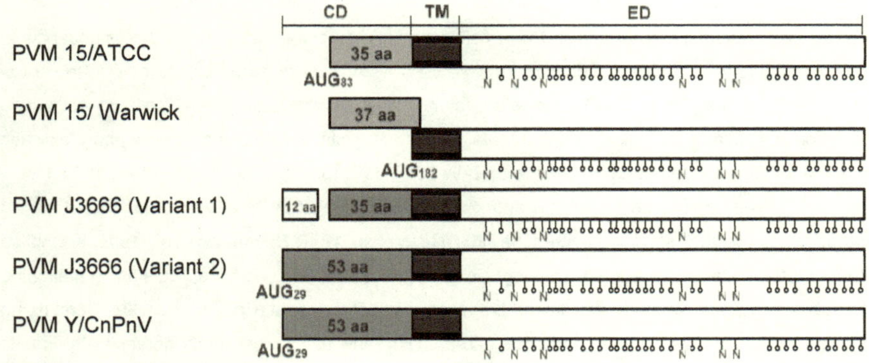

Figure 4: Schematic representation of the G protein of PVM strains.
Diagrammatic representation of the G proteins found in PVM. The possible initiation codons AUG_{29}, AUG_{83} and AUG_{182} of the G mRNA are indicated. The cytoplasmic domain, CT; transmembrane portion, TM; the carboxy-terminus, ED are shown. The six possible N-glycosylation sites and the 32 O-glycosylation sites prediction made with the GlycoEP (Chauhan et al., 2013) are designated with the N and the small circles,

respectively. The upstream open reading frame is shown with the colourless rectangle separated from the main G open reading frame. The slight overlap of the putative CT in PVM 15/Warwick showed that it is not included in the expressed protein. The PVM J3666 (Variant 1) was reported by Randhawa and coworkers (Randhawa et al., 1995) while PVM J3666 (Variant 2) was reported by Krempl and Collins (Krempl and Collins, 2004).

Subsequent analysis with recombinant viruses suggested that the absence of the putative cytoplasmic domain in the G protein was responsible for the attenuated phenotype of the PVM 15/Warwick (Krempl et al., 2007). The effect of the extension of the ORF of the G protein on replication and virulence is yet to be determined but the CnPnV was reported to be somewhat less pathogenic for mice than PVM J3666 (Percopo et al., 2011).

1.7 Propagation of PVM

One of the major challenges that hampered PVM research at the beginning was the absence of suitable *in vitro* culture system. Many cell lines including the standard chicken-embryo fibroblasts were not permissive for efficient virus replication (Tennant and Ward, 1962; Harter and Choppin, 1967). The hamster cell line, BHK-21 clone 13, was the first suitable cell line identified to support high replication of PVM 15 (Harter and Choppin, 1967), yielding viruses with similar morphologically characteristics but somewhat attenuated compared to those produced in the lungs of mice (Harter and Choppin, 1967; Shimonaski and Came, 1970; Weir et al., 1988). Later, BHK-21 cells were reported to support persistent PVM infection without excessive morphological changes to it (Gallaspy et al., 1978). More recently, the virus was reported to replicate efficiently in RAW 264.7 cells, a mouse macrophage-like cell line, in line with previous observations from infected mice (Carthew and Sparrow, 1980; Dyer et al., 2007). However, RAW 264.7 cells cannot be used for propagation of the virus due to contamination with endogenous retroviruses (Hartley et al., 2008).

PVM 15 was reported to grow well and form visible plaques in monkey kidney BS-C-1 cells under certain conditions and virus particles produced in these cells were reported to be comparable to those from BHK-21 cells (Cash et al., 1977). However, later studies showed that BS-C-1 cells do not support isolation of PVM from biological samples containing only few particles neither do they support replication of PVM to high titres, as do BHK-21 cells or RAW 264.7 cells (Schiff, 1976; Miyata et al., 1995; Dyer et al., 2007). The continuous passaging and plaque purification of PVM 15/ATCC in BS-C-1 cells to produce homogenous stock attenuated the virus (Cash et al., 1977; Randhawa et al., 1995; Krempl and Collins, 2004). Hence, to retain the pathogenicity of PVM J3666, the original stock is being maintained by passaging in mouse lungs with limited propagation in BS-C-1 cells (Cook et al., 1998; Dermine and Desmecht, 2012). However, the continuous passaging of PVM 15 in mouse lungs increased its virulence for mice (Horsfall and Hahn, 1940) and this may partially explain the supposed higher virulence of PVM J3666 over PVM 15/Warwick and PVM 15/ATCC (Domachowske et al., 2002; Ellis et al., 2007).

1.8 PVM as a surrogate model of RSV

RSV is the major viral cause of acute lower respiratory tract infections in children worldwide. However, many aspects of its pathogenesis are yet to be unravelled due to unavailability of a suitable animal model. RSV replication is largely restricted in mouse lungs and usually required around 10^6 plaque-forming units to induce moderate clinical symptoms. Furthermore, mice are resistant to reinfection after their first exposure while reinfection is the hallmark of natural infection in children (Derscheid and Ackermann, 2012). The bRSV has a comparable genome arrangement as RSV and bRSV-specific polyclonal antibodies can cross-react with RSV. However, the size of its natural host limits it application as a useful laboratory model (Collins and Crowe, 2006).

PVM shares 52% nucleotide sequence identity with RSV and does not contain the overlap of RSV M2 and L genes nor can PVM-specific antibodies cross-react with RSV (Thorpe and Easton, 2005; Brock et al., 2012). However, studies have shown that PVM and RSV have an identical cell tropism in their respective hosts. In addition, inoculum size of 50 plaque forming units is enough to induce death in mice (Dyer et al., 2012). Furthermore, the PVM genes that have been studied using recombinant viruses appear to be functional homologous of their counterpart in RSV. The PVM-G protein was dispensable in cell culture but it was required for efficient replication in mouse lungs (Krempl et al., 2007) while both the non-structural proteins inhibited induction of type-I and III mouse interferon response (Buchholz et al., 2009; Heinze et al., 2011) as described for RSV, although the mechanism appears to be a little different. Other PVM proteins are thought to have similar biological functions as analogous proteins in RSV due to their similar location in the genome and structural similarities (reviewed by Collins and Crowe, 2006; Easton et al., 2006).

Unlike RSV infections where only a small percentage of infections lead to respiratory ailments in humans, the majority of laboratory mice infected with PVM developed clinical disease with a strong immune response similar to those observed during severe RSV infection. Therefore, PVM is described as a model for the acute severe form of RSV (Rosenberg et al., 2005). Additionally, the patterns of PVM infection in neonatal and adult mice are not considerably different as described for RSV infection with different courses in adult and paediatric patients. However, PVM-infected mice elicit symptoms similar to those observed during human RSV infection (Bem et al., 2011; Dyer et al., 2012). PVM-specific $CD4^+$ and $CD8^+$ T cells recruited into the lungs of infected mice also contributed to pathology as observed in RSV (Claassen et al., 2007; Frey et al., 2008; Walsh et al., 2013). Since the severity of diseases after PVM infection depends on the genetic background of the host (Anh et al., 2006); the strain of the virus (Domachowske et al., 2002); the dose of virus used (Cook et al., 1998; Krempl and Collins, 2004; Bonville et al., 2006); and the age of the mice at the time of infection (Bonville et al., 2007), there is the possibility to combine these factors to obtain models that will mimic RSV infection accurately.

Finally, the development of a reverse genetic system for PVM coupled with the availability of different mouse strains offers the opportunity to study the function of different genes in a natural host-pathogen environment. The observations can then be applied to further our understanding of many unsolved issues in RSV research.

1.9 Translational regulation of protein synthesis by the upstream open reading frame

Upstream open reading frames (uORF) are small ORF coding for 9 to 207 amino acids that precede the main coding ORF of an mRNA. The uORF can be either in frame or out of frame with the main ORF (Calvo et al., 2009). In artificial systems, uORF has been shown to be capable of reducing the translation of the main ORF by up to 80 % (Calvo et al., 2009; Ferreira et al., 2013) and initiate mRNA decay in response to internal or external stimulus (Barbosa et al., 2013).

The recognition of the AUG in an ORF is determined by the translation initiation sequence surrounding the AUG called the Kozak sequence. The optimum Kozak sequence is GCCXCCaugG, taking the the A of the AUG as position +1, adenine or guanine at position -3 (A^{-3} or G^{-3}) and guanine at position +4 (G^{+4}) ensure optimum translation of the ORF containing the AUG (Kozak, 1987). Otherwise, the scanning ribosomes is more likely to slip pass the first AUG of the ORF to the downstream AUG by the leaky scanning method. This usually occurs when uracil or cytosine are found at position -3 or the G^{+4} is changed to another nucleotide (Kozak, 1999). The stronger the Kozak sequence of the uORF, the lower the chance of translating the downstream ORF. Nonetheless, translation of the uORF will occur even in the presence of a weak Kozak sequence, albeit at a lower rate favouring the increased translation of the primary ORF (Meijer and Thomas, 2002; Kozak, 2005). Other factors that can affect the fate of the primary ORF in the presence of an uORF are: length of the uORF, distance between the cap and the AUG of the uORF, the secondary structure of the uORF, the distance between the uORF and the primary ORF, the location and number of stop codons in the uORF (Kozak, 2002; Barbosa et al., 2013).

1.10 Aim and objectives of the book

This project was aimed at understanding the functional contribution of the different G gene variants of PVM J3666 and PVM 15 to replication and virulence. Therefore, experiments were designed:

1. To determine the composition of the G gene variants of quasispecies of PVM J3666 to resolve the discrepancies reported in literature.
2. To generate recombinant viruses PVM based on the strain 15 background containing the G variants of PVM J3666 and subsequently characterize the replication efficiency of the viruses in tissue culture and mice.
3. To compare the replication kinetics of the biological strains of PVM J3666 and PVM 15 in tissue culture to verify if the effect of the G gene structure characterize the behaviour of these strains.

2. Materials and Methods

2.1 Viruses, Mice and Materials

2.1.1 Mice

All mice (Inbred Jackson strain of BALB/c and C57BL/6) used in book were bred at the animal facility of the Institute of Virology and Immunobiology, University of Wuerzburg. All mice were aged 6 - 9 weeks, free of underlying disease and were infected intranasally under anesthesia. Euthanasia at the end of experiments or at humane endpoints was carried out by CO_2 in accordance with the guidelines of the animal ethical committee of the city of Wuerzburg. The experiments were conducted under the approval numbers 87/13 and 30/08.

2.1.2 Viruses

Name	Lab name	Source
rPVM	rPVM1	C. Krempl, VIM Wuerzburg
rPVM-GFP	rPVM1-GFP	C. Krempl, VIM Wuerzburg
rPVM-Gt	rPVM-Gs	C. Krempl, VIM Wuerzburg
rPVM-GFP-Gt		C. Krempl, VIM Wuerzburg
rPVM-ΔG-GFP		C. Krempl, VIM Wuerzburg
rPVM-G_{J3666}65A	rPVM-G_{J3666}65Ap15	generated in section 2.2.8
rPVM-G_{J3666}65U		generated in section 2.2.8
PVM 15/ ATCC		ATCC VR-25
PVM J3666 (G_{J3666}65AU)	PVM J3666	A. Easton, Warwick, UK (AY743909)
PVM J3666 (G_{J3666}65A)	PVM J3666 p15	See sections 2.2.12 and 3.3.1

2.1.3 Cells

Name	Source	Usage
BHK-21	ATCC CCL-10	Virus characterization and propagation
BSR T7/5	Buchholz et al. 1999	Recovery of viable virus from its cDNA
M-CSF L929	M. Lutz, VIM Wuerzburg	Production of M-CSF
MEF cells	Heinze et al. 2011	Virus characterization
RAW 264.7	ATCC TIB-71	Virus characterization
Vero	ATCC CCL-81	Virus quantification

2.1.4 Media for cell culture

Name	Source
Amphotericin B (250 µg/ml)	PAN Biotech, Aidenbach
Dulbecco's MEM (DMEM)	Life Technologies, Darmstadt
Eagle's MEM (EMEM)	Biochrom, Berlin
Foetal calf serum (FCS)	Life Technologies, Darmstadt
G-418 Sulphate (Geneticin), 50 mg/ml	PAA, Austria
Glasgow's MEM (GMEM)	Biochrom, Berlin
L-Glutamine 200 mM	PAN Biotech, Aidenbach
MEM amino acid (50X)	PAN Biotech, Aidenbach
Opti-MEM (reduced serum)	Life Technologies, Darmstadt
Penicillin/Streptomycin (100X)	PAN Biotech, Aidenbach
RPMI-1640	Life Technologies, Darmstadt
Sodium hydrogen carbonate	VIM, Wuerzburg
Sodium pyruvate (100X)	Life Techologies, Darmstadt
Stable Glutamine 200 mM	PAN Biotech, Aidenbach
Trypsin	VIM, Wuerzburg
0.25% Trypsin-EDTA (1X)	Life Technologies, Darmstadt

2.1.5 Plasmids

Name	Source	Usage
p3R1	C. Krempl, VIM Wuerzburg	Cloning of PVM G, F and M2 genes
p3R1-G_{J3666}65A	See section 2.2.2	Cloning of PVM G, F and M2 genes
p3R1-G_{J3666}65U	See section 2.2.2	Cloning of PVM G, F and M2 genes
pGEM 3Zf(+)	Promega, Mannheim	Cloning of PVM J3666 fragment
pPVM	C. Krempl, VIM Wuerzburg	Cloning of full-length plasmid and virus rescue
pPVM -G_{J3666}65A	See section 2.2.2	Cloning of full-length plasmid and virus rescue
pPVM-G_{J3666}65U	See section 2.2.2	Cloning of full-length plasmid and virus rescue
pTM L	C. Krempl, VIM Wuerzburg	Support plasmid for virus rescue
pTM M2-1	C. Krempl, VIM Wuerzburg	Support plasmid for virus rescue
pTM N	C. Krempl, VIM Wuerzburg	Support plasmid for virus rescue
pTM P	C. Krempl, VIM Wuerzburg	Support plasmid for virus rescue
pUC19	NEB, Ipswich England	Cloning of PVM J3666 fragment

2.1.6 Competent cell and media

Chemically competent *Escherichia coli* (K12 strain, NEB-10) were used for all cloning experiments described in this book. The bacteria were grown at 32°C and transformed as described in section 2.2.6.

SOC	NEB, Ipswich England
Lysogeny Broth (LB) medium	10 g tryptone extract 10 g NaCl 5 g yeast extract Bring to 1 litre with H_2O and autoclave
LB Agar	LB broth 15 g agar Bring to 1 litre with H_2O and autoclave

2.1.7 DNA and RNA modifying enzymes

Name	Source
DNaseI, RNase free	Thermo Scientific, St. Leon-Roth
GoTaq® DNA polymerase	Promega, Mannheim
iTaq™ Universal SYBR Green supermix	Bio-Rad, Munich
Phusion® HF DNA polymerase	NEB, Ipswich England
Rapid DNA dephos and ligation kit	Roche, Mannheim
RevertAid™ H minus reverse transcriptase	Thermo Scientific, St. Leon-Roth
RiboLock™ RNase inhibitor	Thermo Scientific, St. Leon-Roth
RNase A, DNase and protein free	Thermo Scientific, St. Leon-Roth
RNase H	NEB, Ipswich England

2.1.8 Primers

Name	Orientation and sequence (5' – 3')
Fw primer with Acc65I	Fw- *CACACA*<u>GGTACC</u>TTGATAGTGTGGAGCAG
Rs primer with Acc65I	Rs- *CACACA*<u>GGTACC</u>AAGAATCAAACCGAGGAAC
J3666 G AgeI fw	Fw- *ACACAC*<u>ACCGGT</u>AGGATAAGTACTATCCTATTG
[b]18s RNA Fw	Fw- TCAAGAACGAAAGTCGGAGGTT
[b]18s RNA Rs	Rs- GGACATCTAAGGGCATCACAG
[a]PVM F Fw	Fw- GACCGACCTGATTTACCT
[a]PVM F Rs	Rs- CACCATTGTTTAAGCCCA
PVM G Fw	Fw- GCACATACACTACACCAG
PVM G Rs	Rs- GCAGACCAGTTACATTGAC
[a]PVM N Fw	Fw - AGGACACTCGGCATGTTCTT
[a]PVM N Rs	Rs- GTCCTTGAGCTGTGTGTCCA
PVM 4039	Fw- ACACAGCACAACAACCACCG
6857	Fw- GTCACGACGTTGTAAAACGAC
6858	Rs- CAGGAAACAGCTATGACCATG
6993	Fw- CACCACAGAGCAAGGGAC
6994	Fw- AGAGGTTACCACCCTTTC

6995	Fw- CCTAAGTCCTCAGGCTTAC
6996	Rs- CTTGTTGTTAAACCTAGG
6997	Rs- GATGTTCAGGACCTGGAG
6998	Rs- CACAAACTGCCACAGCAGC
7926	Rs- TCCACTGCACTACTATAGATTGC

The italicized and underlined sequences were extra nucleotides added to aid restriction and to artificially introduced restriction sites, respectively. All primers were purchased from Biomers Ulm, Germany. Source: [a]Buchholz et al., 2009; [b]Marino et al., 2003.

2.1.9 Restriction enzymes

Enzyme	Source
Acc65I	Thermo Scientific, St. Leon-Roth
AccI	NEB, Ipswich England
AgeI-HF	NEB, Ipswich England
BstBI	NEB, Ipswich England
HindIII	Thermo Scientific, St. Leon-Roth
NdeI	NEB, Ipswich England
PacI	NEB, Ipswich England

2.1.10 Purified antibodies and antisera

Name	Source	Dilution
Anti-mouse CD11b	BD Pharmingen, Heidelberg	1:400
Anti-mouse CD16/32	ebioscience, San Diego, USA	1:400
Anti-mouse F4/80	ebioscience, San Diego, USA	1:200
Biotinylated goat anti-rabbit IgG (H+L)	Thermo Scientific, St. Leon-Roth	1:5000
Goat anti-mouse IgG, (H+L) HRP	Dako, Darmstadt	1:3000
Goat anti-rabbit IgG, (H+L) HRP	Millipore, Darmstadt	1:3000
LIVE/DEAD® fixable violet dead cell stain	Life Technologies, Darmstadt	
Mouse anti-rPVM-GFP sera (1000 PFU)	VIM, Wuerzburg	1:300
Rabbit anti-PVM G	Dr Krempl, VIM Wuerzburg	1:3000
Streptavidin-HRP	BD Pharmingen, Heidelberg	1:2000

2.1.11 Commercial kits

Name	Source
QIAGEN® Plasmid Maxi Kit	Qiagen, Hilden
QIAGEN® Plasmid Midi Kit	Qiagen, Hilden
QIAprep® Spin Miniprep Kit	Qiagen, Hilden

QIAquick® Gel electrophoresis kit	Qiagen, Hilden
QIAquick® PCR purification kit	Qiagen, Hilden
QIAshredder™	Qiagen, Hilden
RNeasy® mini kit	Qiagen, Hilden
Roti® Quant Universal reagent 1 and 2	Roth, Karlsruhe
WesternBright™ chemiluminescence substrate	Biozym, Oldendorf

2.1.12 Laboratory instruments

Name	Source
ABI 7300/7500 Real time PCR System	Life technologies, Darmstadt
Biofuge pico Centrifuge	Heraeus, Sepatech
Biometra Tpersonal thermocycler	Biometra, Goettingen
Centrifuge 5415R	Eppendorf. Hamburg
Chemical hood	Wesemann and Striepe, Ulm
Electrophoresis gel jet imager	Intas, Goettingen
Electrophoresis power supply	Consort, Belgium
Eppendorf Mastercycler personal	Eppendorf, Hamburg
Flow cytometer (LSR II and FACSCalibur)	BD Biosceinces, Heidelberg
Fridge / freezers	Bosch, Gerligen
Fridge / freezers	Liebherr, Biberach
Fujifilm intelligent dark box LAS 3000	Fujifilm, Dusseldorf
Gilson pipettes (P2, P10, P20, P100, P200 and P1000)	Gilson, Limburg-Offheim
HLC heating-thermomixer MHR 11	Dibitas AG, Pforzheim
Hotplate stirrer (I-81)	Labinco BV, Netherlands
Ice Maker	Scotsmann, Italy
Incubator (normal and CO_2)	Heraeus electronic
Inverted fluorescence microscope (DMIRE2)	Leica, Solms
Inverted light microscope (TS100)	Nikon, Dusseldorf
Megafuge 1.0R centrifuge	Heraeus Sepatech
Multichannel pipette	Brand, Wertheim
Nalgene Cryo 1°C freezing container	Nalgene, USA
NanoDrop 2000 spectrophometer	Peqlab, Erlangen
Safety hood (Class II Type A/B3)	Nuaire, USA
Shaker	Froebel Labortechnik, Lindau
Shaker with incubator	Certomat, Goettingen
Vortex machine	Heidolph, Schwabach
Water bath	Memmert, Schwabach

2.1.13 Chemicals

Name	Source
2-Amino-2-hydroxymethyl-propane-1,3-diol (Tris-base)	AppliChem, Darmstadt
2-Mercaptoethanol	Merck, Darmstadt
3,3',4,4'-Tetraamino-diphenyl (DAB)	AppliChem, Darmstadt
Acetic Acid	AppliChem, Darmstadt
Agar agar	AppliChem, Darmstadt
Agarose	Biozym, Oldendorf
Albumin Fraction V, pH 7 (BSA)	Roth, Karlsruhe
Amphotericin B, 50X	PAN Biotech, Aidenbach
Ampicillin sodium salt	AppliChem, Darmstadt
Aprotinin	AppliChem, Darmstadt
Bromophenol blue	AppliChem, Darmstadt
Dimethyl sulphate oxide	AppliChem, Darmstadt
EDTA solution pH 8.0	AppliChem, Darmstadt
Ethanol	AppliChem, Darmstadt
Fetal bovine Serum (FCS)	PAA, Pasching
Glucose	AppliChem, Darmstadt
Glycerol	AppliChem, Darmstadt
Glycine	AppliChem, Darmstadt
HEPES	AppliChem, Darmstadt
Hydrochloric acid (2N)	Roth, Karlsruhe
Isoflurane	Essex Tierarznei, Essen
Isopropanal	AppliChem, Darmstadt
Lipofectamine® 2000	Life Technologies, Darmstadt
Magnesium sulphate (anhydrous)	AppliChem, Darmstadt
Methanol	Roth, Karlsruhe
Methylcellulose	Roth, Karlsruhe
Phenol	Roth, Karlsruhe
Potassium acetate	AppliChem, Darmstadt
Potassium chloride	AppliChem, Darmstadt
Potassium hydroxide	AppliChem, Darmstadt
Protease inhibitor cocktail tablet	Roche, Mannheim
Random primers (400 ng /µl)	Qiagen, Hilden
Rotiphorese gel 40	Roth, Karlsruhe
Sodium acetate	AppliChem, Darmstadt
Sodium azide	AppliChem, Darmstadt
Sodium Chloride (>99.8%)	Roth, Karlsruhe
Sodium dodecyl sulphate	Roth, Karlsruhe
Sodium hydroxide	AppliChem, Darmstadt

Sucrose	AppliChem, Darmstadt
Synthetic oligonucleotides (primers)	Biomers GmbH, Ulm
Taurocholic acid	Sigma Aldrich, Munich
Terralin disinfectant	Schulke and Mayer
Trichloromethane	Roth, Karlsruhe
Tris-HCl	AppliChem, Darmstadt
TRIzol® LS reagent	Life Technologies, Darmstadt
Trypan blue	AppliChem, Darmstadt
Tryptone	AppliChem, Darmstadt
Tween 20	Roth, Karlsruhe
Yeast Extract	AppliChem, Karlsruhe
α-amino-n-caproic acid	Sigma Aldrich, Munich

2.1.14 Plastics wares and other consumables

Name	Source
Tubes	
0.5 ml	Sarstedt, Nuembrecht
1.5 ml and 2ml safe-lock tubes	Eppendorf, Hamburg
2 ml cyro tubes	Greiner Bio-One, Frickenhausen
5 ml FACS tubes	BD, Heidelberg
5 ml tissue culture tubes	Falcon, USA
15 ml	Greiner Bio-One, Frickenhausen
50 ml	Greiner Bio-One, Frickenhausen
PCR tubes	Brand, Wertheim
Cell scrapper	Biochrom, Berlin
Plates	
6-well flat bottom	Greiner Bio-One, Frickenhausen
12-well flat bottom	Greiner Bio-One, Frickenhausen
24-well flat bottom	Greiner Bio-One, Frickenhausen
96-well U-bottom	Greiner Bio-One, Frickenhausen
Cell culture flask	
50 ml	Greiner Bio-One, Frickenhausen
250 ml	Greiner Bio-One, Frickenhausen
800 ml	Greiner Bio-One, Frickenhausen

2.1.15 Solutions and buffers

Protein analysis and Western blotting

2X Laemmli buffer	10 ml 1 M Tris pH 6.8 20 ml 10% SDS 10 ml 100% glycerol 10 ml H_2O 1 tablet of proteinase inhibitors
Resolving gel (8 %)	2.67 ml 30% polyacrylamide 2.5 ml 1.5 ml of Tris pH 8.8 100 µl 10% SDS 100 µl 10% APS 6 µl TEMED 4.63 ml H_2O
Stacking gel (5 %) gel	850 µl 30% polyacrylamide 625 µl 1ml of Tris pH 6.8 50 µl 10% SDS 50 µl 10% APS 5 µl TEMED 3.4 ml H_2O
Running buffer (10X)	10 g SDS 30 g Tris 144 g Glycine Bring to 1 litre with H_2O
Blotting buffer 1 (Anode 1, pH 10.4)	300 ml 1M Tris base (pH 10.4) 200 ml 100% ethanol Bring to 1 litre with H_2O
Blotting buffer 2 (Anode 2, pH 10.4)	25 ml 1 M Tris base (pH 10.4) 200 ml 100% ethanol Bring to 1 litre with H_2O
Blotting buffer 3 (Cathode, pH 9.4)	25 ml 1 M Tris base (pH 9.4) 200 ml 100% ethanol 5.2 g ε-aminocaproic acid Bring to 1 litre with H_2O
Phosphate buffer saline (PBS) for routine use	In-house
PBS with Tween 20 (PBST)	PBS with 0.05% (v/v) Tween 20

Buffer for plasmid preparation

Miniprep resuspension buffer (Add 100 µl of RNase A /10 ml of buffer, store at 4°C)	2.25 g Glucose 2 ml 0.5 M EDTA (pH 8.0) 2.5 ml 1 M Tris-HCl Bring to 250 ml with H_2O
Minprep lysis buffer	2 g NaOH 2.5 g SDS Bring to 250 ml with H_2O
Miniprep neutralization buffer	29.445 g potassium acetate 11.5 ml acetic acid Bring to 250 ml with H_2O
Salt buffer	8 g NaOH (2 M) 4 ml 0.5 M EDTA (pH 8.0) 5 ml 1 M Tris (pH 7.5) Bring to 100 ml with H_2O

Gel electrophoresis

50X Tris-acetate EDTA (TAE) buffer	242 g Tris base 57.1 ml of 100% acetic acid 100 ml 0.5 M EDTA (pH 8.0) Bring to 1 litre with H_2O
Agarose gel (1%)	1 g agarose 100 ml H_2O 100 µl 0.07% Ethidium bromide
DNA Loading buffer (10X)	0.0125 g bromophenol blue 200 µl 0.5 M EDTA (pH 8.0) 3.9 ml 100% glycerol 500 µl 10% SDS Bring to 10 ml with H_2O

Tissue culture

Buffer for virus stablility (pH 7.5)	12.04 g MgSO4 (1 M) 11.91 g HEPES (0.5 M) Bring to 100 ml with H_2O

2.1.16 Computer software

Software	Source
Adobe illustrator (CS3)	Adobe systems Inc, USA
AIDA (v 3.20.116)	Raytest GmbH, Berlin
EndNote X7	Thomson Reuters, USA
FlowJo (v 8.0)	TreeStar Inc, USA
GraphPad prism 4.0	GraphPad, USA
ImageJ	NIH, USA
Lasergene 11.0	DNAStar, USA
Mendeley	London, UK
Microsoft windows and office	Microsoft, USA
MEGA6	megasoftware.net

2.2 Methods

2.2.1 Cells

Vero cells were grown in Eagle's minimum essential medium (MEM) supplemented with 10% FCS and 2mM L-Glutamine. BHK-21 cells and BSR-T7/5 constitutively expressing T7 polymerase were maintained in Glasgow's MEM containing 10% FCS, 2mM stable glutamine and 2% MEM amino acid. The BSR-T7/5 cells were treated with 0.5 µg/ml of Geneticin (PAA) after every other passage to ensure continuous expression of the T7 polymerase. RAW 264.7 cells were grown in Dulbecco's MEM (DMEM) supplemented with 1% sodium pyruvate, 2.6% sodium hydrogen carbonate, 10% FCS, 1% amphotericin B and 1% penicillin-streptomycin. Mouse embryonic fibroblast (MEF) cells derived from C57BL/6 and C57BL/6.IFNAR$^{-/-}$ mice were maintained in DMEM supplemented with 10% FCS, 2 mM L-glutamine and 2.6% sodium hydrogen carbonate and were used below 10 passages. M-CSF L929 cells were maintained in RPMI-1640 supplemented with 10% FCS, 1% amphotericin B, 1% penicillin/streptomycin and 1% amino acids for maximum of five passages per time. Bone marrow-derived macrophages were maintained in RPMI-1640 containing 20% M-CSF, 10% FCS, 1% HEPES, 1% sodium pyruvate, 1% amphotericin B and 1% penicillin/streptomycin). All cells were confirmed to be mycoplasma free before use and were passaged less than 30 times unless otherwise stated.

2.2.2 Virus propagation

The PVM J3666 stock used in this book was prepared from BHK-21 cells inoculated with lung homogenate from BALB/c mice infected with PVM strain J3666 (AY743909) originally provided by Dr. Andrew Easton of the University of Warwick, England. PVM J3666, PVM 15, and recombinant pneumonia virus of mice (rPVM) and its derivatives were propagated in BHK-21 cells.at an initial multiplicity of infection (MOI) of 0.01 PFU/cells. Confluent layers of BHK-21 cells were infected with appropriate volume of virus suspension diluted in minimal amount (7.5 ml for T75 flask or 10 ml for T175 flask) of GMEM infection medium (GMEM containing 5% FCS, 2mM stable glutamine and 2% MEM amino acid, 1% amphotericin B and 1% penicillin-streptomycin) for 3 hours with intermittent rocking at 32°C. After the initial adsorption, the volume was doubled and incubation was continued for 7 days with a change of medium on days 2 and 4 postinfection to ensure optimum yield. On day 7, the infected cells were scrapped into the supernatant followed by addition of 10% (v/v) virus preservative and centrifugation (800 xg and 10 minutes at 4°C). Thereafter, two-third of the supernatant was transferred into tube and kept on ice while the pellet was homogenized in the remainder supernatant by three freeze-thaw cycles and vortexing to release the cell-bound virus particles. The homogenized sample was clarified by centrifugation at 800 xg for 10 minutes and 4°C and combined with the other supernatant on ice before aliquots were prepared and snap frozen in liquid nitrogen. All viruses were stored at -80°C.

To select a single virus population from the mixed PVM J3666 population, the PVM J3666 stock was sequentially passaged in BHK-21 cells or RAW 264.7 cells seeded in 6-well plate as described above. Total cellular RNA was collected from cellular debris collected after infection as described in 2.2.5.

2.2.3 Virus quantification by plaque assay

Virus titres were determined by plaque assay on Vero cells seeded in 24-well plates. The cells were infected with a 10-fold serial dilution of virus suspension in EMEM for three hours with intermittent shaking. Thereafter the inoculum was removed and overlaid with 0.8% methylcellulose for 6 days at 32°C. The plaques were twice fixed with 80% ice-cold methanol for one hour and stained with rabbit polyclonal antibody against PVM-G. Bound antibodies were detected with a biotinylated goat anti-rabbit IgG, followed by amplification with streptavidin coupled with horseradish peroxidase (HRP). Colour development was made with 3,3'-diaminobenzidine tetrahydrochloride (DAB) substrate and hydrogen peroxide. For virus lacking the G gene, GFP-positive plaques were counted by using an inverted fluorescence microscope (Leica DM IRE2, Solms). The titres of the tested viruses were determined using the formula:

$$\left(\frac{(mean\ plaque\ count\ (PFU)}{0.15\ ml}\right) X \frac{1}{dilution\ factor}, PFU = plaque - forming\ unit$$

Plaque counts ranging between 20 and 200 per well were used, as lower and higher plaque counts were often irreproducible.

2.2.4 Replication kinetics in tissue culture

Multicycle or single-cycle replication kinetics was performed with confluent monolayers of BHK-21 cells or mouse embryonic fibroblasts or RAW 264.7 cells at desired MOI. The cells were infected as described in section 2.2.2 except that a washing step with PBS pre-warmed to 37°C was included after the initial virus adsorption to remove unbound virus particles and this time point was recorded as day 0. With the exception of RAW 264.7 cells, where only cell-free viruses were collected during some experiments, cell-bound and cell-free viruses were collected at the different time points. Ten percent (v/v) buffer containing 50 mM HEPES and 100 mM $MgSO_4$ was added to the harvested culture for stabilization, followed by vigorous vortexing for 3 minutes to release cell-bound particles and centrifugation in a tabletop centrifuge (8,000 xg for 10 minutes at 4°C) to remove cellular debris. Aliquots of the supernatant were prepared, frozen with nitrogen, and quantified as shown in 2.2.3.

2.2.5 Amplification of a PVM J3666 fragment spanning M to F genes (J3666-MSHGF)

Isolation of total RNA from BHK-21-infected PVM J3666-MSHGF

Total cellular RNA was collected from BHK-21 cells in a 6-well plate infected with PVM J3666 at an MOI of 0.01 PFU/cell after 48 hours using TRIzol LS® reagent (Life technologies, Darmstadt) as described by the manufacturer. The obtained RNA pellet was dissolved in 40 µl DEPC water and quantified using NanoDrop 2000 (Thermo Scientific, Leon-Roth).

Generation of J3666-MSHGF cDNA

The total cellular RNA was reversed transcribed into complementary DNA (cDNA) with random primers and RevertAid™ H minus reverse transcriptase (Thermo Scientific) as shown in table 1. After inactivation of the transcriptase at 70°C for 10 minutes, 2 U of RNase H (NEB, Ipswich England) was added per tube to destroy the RNA in the RNA-DNA hybrid. The desired PVM J3666 PCR fragment (J3666-MSHGF, 2517 bp) covering from nucleotide 3708 through 6195 of the PVM genome corresponding to 406 bases in the M gene, the complete SH and G genes, and 314 nucleotides of the F gene was prepared with the Phusion DNA polymerase (NEB) from the single-stranded cDNA using the conditions in table 2. The PCR product was electrophoresed in 1% agarose gel, J3666-MSHGF fragment was excised and purified by a QIAquick® gel extraction kit (Qiagen, Hilden).

Table 1: Typical setup for cDNA generation

Reagent	Volume	
RNA (total RNA (≤ 5 µg) or viral RNA (≤ 500 ng)	X µl	
Random primer (400 ng/µl, Qiagen)	0.5 µl	
H_2O	add to 12.5 µl	
Addition of master mix		
dNTP mix (10 mM)	2 µl	
5x RT buffer	4 µl	
RNase inhibitor (40 U/µl)	0.5 µl	
RevertAid™ H minus reverse transcriptase (200 U/µl)	1 µl	
Final volume	20 µl	
Program	**Temperature**	**Time**
Denaturation of RNA secondary structure	65°C	5 min
Hold	4°C	at least for 2 min
Addition of master mix		
Primer annealing	25°C	10 min
Extension	50°C	60 min
Inactivation of RT enzyme	70°C	10 min
Hold	4°C	pause
Removal of RNA in RNA:DNA hybrid	37°C	20 min
Hold	4°C	pause

Table 2: Gene-specific amplification of RT-product (J3666-MSHGF)

Reagent	Volume (final concentration)		
Reaction buffer (5X)	10 µl		
dNTP mix (10 mM)	1 µl (200 µM)		
Acc65I Fw	2.5 µl (0.5 µM)		
Acc65I RS	2.5 µl (0.5 µM)		
Phusion polymerase	0.5 µl (0.02 U)		
PVM J3666 cDNA	2 µl		
H_20	ad 50 µl		
Program	**Temperature**	**Time**	**Cycle**
Initial denaturation	98°C	2 min	1 X
Denaturation	98°C	10 sec	35 X
Annealing	60°C	15 sec	

Extension	72°C	30 sec /kb	
Final extension	72°C	8 min	1 X
Hold	4°C	pause	

Note: Annealing temperature was calculated with the NEB Tm calculator: https://www.neb.com/tools-and-resources/interactive-tools/tm-calculator (accessed 26.07.11).

Nucleotide sequencing of J3666-MSHGF fragments

The nucleotide composition of the purified J3666-MSHGF fragment was determined with the BigDye terminator ready reaction kit (v1.1 Applied Biosystems, Massachusetts USA) and a genetic analyser (ABI PRISM 310, Applied Biosytems) based on primers 6993, 6994, 6995, 6996, 6997 and 6998 as described in table 3. The consensus sequence of the fragment was derived from the alignment of the electrophoretograms with the SeqMan program (v 11.0, DNASTAR, Madison-Wisconsin USA).

Table 3: Sequencing reaction of J3666-MSHGF fragment

Reagent	Volume	Final concentration	
DNA	x µl	≈20 ng	
Primer (10 pmol/µl)	0.5 µl	5 pmol /µl	
2.5X Tris buffer	1 µl		
BigDye Terminator v1.1	1 µl		
H_2O	ad 5 µl		
Program	**Temperature**	**Time**	**Cycle**
Denaturation	96°C	20 sec	24 X
Annealing	50°C	20 sec	
Extension	60°C	4 min	
Hold	4°C	Pause	

2.2.6 Molecular cloning of J3666-MSHGF

Digestion and ligation of J3666-MSHGF and plasmid vector

One microgram of the purified J3666-MSHGF fragment and 2 µg of vector (pUC19 or pGEM-3Zf(+)) were separately digested overnight with 10 U/µg of *Acc65I* at 37°C followed by separation on 1% agarose gel electrophoresis. The desired insert and vector fragments were excised from the gel, purified by the Qiaquick gel extraction kit (Qiagen). The purified vector was dephosphorylated with alkaline phosphatase (Roche, Mannheim) as shown in table 4 and then ligated with the insert as described in table 5 using the Roche DNA dephos and ligation kit (Roche).

Table 4: Dephosphorylation of vector ends

Reagent	Volume	Final concentration
Vector DNA	X µl	1 µg
rAPid Alkaline Phosphatase buffer (10X)	2 µl	1X
rAPid Alkaline Phosphatase	1 µl	1 U
Deionized water	ad 20 µl	
Final Volume	20 µl	

Table 5: Ligation of dephosphorylated vector and insert

Reagents	Volume	Final concentration
Dephosphorylated Vector DNA	X µl	50 ng
Insert DNA	X µl	150 ng
DNA dilution buffer (5X)	2 µl	1X
Distilled water	ad 10 µl	
Thorough mixing of all components		
T4 DNA ligation buffer (2X)	10 µl	1X
T4 ligase	1 µl	5U
Thorough mixing and incubation at room temperature for 40 minutes		

Transformation of ligated DNA into competent cells

The ligated product was transformed into competent *E. coli* (NEB 10-beta). Three microliters of the ligated DNA were diluted with 2 µl of sterile water and transferred into a 5 ml tube containing 20 µl of competent cells on ice. The tube was gently flicked to mix the samples, incubated on ice for 30 minutes before the cells were transferred to 42°C for 30 seconds and kept on ice for another 5 minutes. Thereafter, 250 µl of SOC outgrowth medium was added to the sample, followed by incubation at 37°C with shaking at 200 rpm for 1 hour. Subsequently, 50 µl of the outgrowth medium was plated on LB agar containing 100 µg/ml and the plate were incubated at 32°C until colonies were visible.

Isolation of plasmid DNA (mini-preparation)

Distinct colonies of transformed bacteria were used to inoculate freshly prepared 3 ml of LB medium containing 100 µg of ampicillin, followed by incubation at 37°C for 14 hours. The bacteria were collected at 13,000 rpm for 1 minute and the pellet was dissolved in 250 µl of resuspension buffer by vortexing, followed by lysis with 250 µl of the lysis buffer. After 4 minutes of incubation at 25°C, 350 µl of neutralization buffer was added to the tube to stop lysis, which was achieved by vigorously inverting the tube. The lysate was incubated on ice for 10 minutes to precipitate the DNA, clarified by centrifugation at 13, 000 rpm for 15 minutes in a tabletop centrifuge and the supernatant was decanted into a new tube. Afterwards, 450 µl of isopropanol was added to the supernatant, mixed with vortex for 15 seconds to precipitate the plasmid DNA that was collected at 13,000 rpm for 20 minutes. The DNA was washed with 500 µl of 70% ethanol and recollected at 13,000 rpm for 15 minutes. The DNA was recovered with 40 µl of water after all traces of ethanol had evaporated. The orientation and size of the plasmid DNAs were determined by analytic digestion using *HindIII* (5 U per 20 µl) restriction endonuclease for 1 hour at 37°C. The digested plasmid was separated on 1% agarose gel, stained with ethidium bromide and visualized under ultraviolet light (Figure 5).

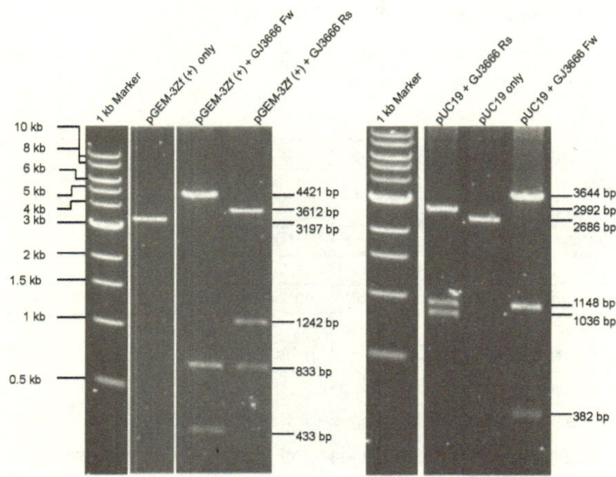

Figure 5: Confirmation of size and orientation of cloned PVM J3666 insert.
Between 0.5 - 1 µg of the each plasmid was digested with 7 *U* of *Hind*III and separated on 1 % agarose gel containing 1% (v/v) of 0.07% ethidium bromide in 1X TAE buffer at 8 V/cm for 1.5 hours. The image was recorded under ultraviolet light. The sizes of the digested fragments: pGEM-3Zf (+) clones (21 Fw and 11 Rs) and pUC19 (7 Fw and 6 Rs) were confirmed with the 1 kb ladder (NEB).

Sequencing of the J3666-MSHGF insert in the plasmid vector

The protocol in section 2.2.5 was used to determine the sequence composition of the portion of interest in the cloned J3666-MSHGF insert from plasmids isolated above. The M gene portion was amplified with primers PVM 4039 and 6858; the SH gene with primers 6857 and 6998; the G gene with primers 6993, 6994, 6997, and 6998; and the F gene with primer 7926. Mutations found in only one clone were ignored during the assembly of the consensus sequence.

2.2.7 Generation of pPVM-G_{J3666}65A and pPVM-G_{J3666}65U plasmids

Preparation of G_{J3666} inserts for cloning into pPVM plasmid

The J3666-MSHGF insert in pGEM-3Zf(+) containing the appropriate G_{J3666}65A or G_{J3666}65U variant was amplified with Phusion DNA polymerase (NEB) using a forward primer that added an *AgeI* site upstream of the G gene and a reverse primer that bound 256 bp downstream of the G gene within the F gene as shown in section 2.2.5. The G_{J3666}65A-PCR and G_{J3666}65U-PCR fragments were prepared using the reagent setup in table 5 and conditions listed in table 6.

Table 6: Amplification of G_{J3666} inserts from J3666-MSHGF fragment cloned into pGEM-3Zf(+)

Template	Forward primer	Reverse primer	Annealing temperature	Amplicon size
J3666-MSHGF in pGEM 3Zf (+)	J3666 G AgeI Fw	7926	60°	1610 bp

The G_{J3666}65A-PCR and G_{J3666}65U-PCR fragments were electrophoresed in 1% agarose gel, excised and purified by a QIAquick® gel extraction kit (Qiagen, Hilden). Later, the fragments were sequenced to confirm their composition as described in section 2.5.

Insertion of G_{J3666} inserts into pPVM to produce pPVM-G_{J3666}65A and pPVM-G_{J3666}65U

pPVM is a plasmid containing the full-length antigenomic cDNA of PVM 15 (Krempl et al., 2007). pPVM was prepared from assembly of five subgenomic plasmids. To produce pPVM-G_{J3666}65U and pPVM-G_{J3666}65A containing the PVM J3666-G gene variants in place of PVM 15-G gene, the subgenomic plasmid, p3R1, enclosing the G, F and M2 genes, flanked by unique *AgeI* and *BstBI* restriction sites before the G gene and at the end of M2 gene, respectively, was employed. p3R1-G_{J3666}65U was prepared by replacing 931 nucleotides in the G gene of p3R1 with equivalent portion from purified G_{J3666}65U-PCR fragment prepared above via *AgeI* restriction site before the G gene and unique *AvrII* restriction site within the G gene. Whereas p3R1-G_{J3666}65A was generated by replacing the entire G gene and the first 155 nt of the F gene in p3R1 with equivalent portion in G_{J3666}65A-PCR fragment via the *AgeI* restriction site and sole *NdeI* restriction site in the adjacent F gene. Afterward, the new p3R1-G_{J3666}65U and p3R1-G_{J3666}65A were reintroduced into the full-length pPVM backbone via via the *AgeI* and *BstBI* restriction sites to produce pPVM-G_{J3666}65U and pPVM-G_{J3666}65A, respectively. Large quantities of the plasmids were prepared using the QIAprep® spin maxiprep kit (Qiagen) and purified by phenol-chloroform extraction to remove residual proteins.

2.2.8 Isolation of rPVM-G_{J3666}65U and rPVM-G_{J3666}65A from plasmids

pPVM-G_{J3666}65U and pPVM-G_{J3666}65A and a cocktail of support plasmids expressing the subunits of the PVM polymerase (N, L, P and M2-1 proteins) under the control of T7 polymerase were transfected into confluent BSR T7/5 cells as described by Krempl and co-workers (Krempl et al., 2007). A Confluent monolayer of BSR T7/5 cells in a well of a 6-well plate (35-mm diameter) were twice washed with 2 ml of Opti-MEM without FCS, incubated with another 2 ml for 1 hour at 37°C. While the incubation elapsed, the plasmid mix and lipofectamine mix were prepared as shown in table 7. The prepared plasmid mix and lipofectamine mix were combined, mixed by pipetting, and incubated at room temperature for 20 minutes to get the transfection mix. Thereafter, 1,600 µl of fresh Opti-MEM was added to the transfection mix and gently mixed with a single-use 2 ml glass pipette. The supernatants in the wells were removed and each well was overlaid with 1 mL of the diluted transfection mix. The cells were then incubated overnight at 37°C and 5% CO_2.

Table 7: Set-up for transfection of full-length plasmid DNA

Plasmid mix				
Reagents	Test plasmid (2X)		Control plasmid	
	Conc.	Volume	Conc.	Volume
Full-length plasmid (0.5 µg /µL)	10 µg	20 µl		
pTM pvmN (0.5 µg /µL)	4 µg	8 µl		
pTM pvm P (0.5 µg /µL)	4 µg	8 µl		
pTM pvmM2-1 (0.5 µg /µL)	2 µg	4 µl		
pTM pvmL (0.5 µg /µL)	2 µg	4 µl		
pTM GFP (0.5 µg /µL)			4 µg	8 µl
Opti-MEM (reduced serum)		156 µl		92 µl
Final volume		200 µl		100 µl
Lipofectamine mix (1 µg of DNA: 3 µl of Lipofectamine 2000)				
	Full-length plasmid		Control plasmid	
Lipofectamine	66 µl		12 µl	
Opti-MEM (reduced serum)	144 µl		88 µl	
Final volume	200 µl		100 µl	
Incubate at room temperature for 5 minutes				

After overnight incubation, the transfection mix was aseptically removed by suction and the cells were washed two times with 2 ml of GMEM infection medium and then overlaid with fresh 2 ml of GMEM infection medium. The plates were incubated for 4 days at 32°C, 5% CO_2. The level of GFP expression in the control well was used to predict the efficiency of the transfection. On day 5 post-transfection, 500 µl of the supernatant was removed for virus titration (see 2.2.3) while the cells were scrapped into the remaining supernatant and co-cultivated with BHK-21 cells (1.5 x 10^6 cells) in a T25 flask to produce the first virus passage. Thereafter, the viruses were propagated in BHK-21 cells with an initial MOI of 0.01 PFU/cell until a useable titre was reached at passage 3 (see 2.2.2). Total RNA was collected from the cellular debris after virus harvest at the third passage was used to produce an amplicon similar to J3666-MSHGF and the sequence composition of the fragment was determined by as described in 2.2.5.

2.2.9 Western blot analysis of protein

Total cellular and virus lysates were separated on 8 % SDS containing polyacrylamide gels and transferred onto a nitrocellulose membrane. After electroblotting, the transferred proteins were detected with antiserum from convalescent mice that recovered from rPVM infection.

Preparation of total cellular and virus lysates

Total cellular lysates were prepared from three wells of BHK-21 cells in 35-mm plate infected at MOI of 0.1 PFU/cell with recombinant viruses or biological isolates for 96 hours. The cells were washed twice with and collected by gentle scraping into 1ml ice-cold PBS. The cells were pelleted at 300 rpm for 7 minutes, dissolved in 100 µl of ice-cold PBS and lysed with equal volume of 2X Laemelli buffer (Laemmli, 1970). The lysates were clarified at 13,000 rpm for 2 minutes at 4°C using a cell shredder and the total protein yields were quantified with the Roti Universal quant kit (Roth, Karlsruhe).

To prepare virus lysates, virus particles from 650 ml flask of BHK-21 cells infected at MOI of 1 PFU/cell with the desired viruses were harvested after 48 hours as shown in section 2.2.3. The virus particles in the supernatant were pelleted at 26,000g for 90 minutes at 4°C through a 4 ml 30% sucrose (w/w) gradient. The pelleted virus particles were washed twice with ice-cold PBS, dissolved in 200 µl of ice-cold PBS and lysed with 200 µl of 2X Laemelli buffer (4% SDS, 20% glycerol and 120 mM Tris, pH 6.8). The lysates were clarified with a cell shredder at 13,000 rpm for 2 minutes at 4°C.

One-dimensional SDS-PAGE

Thirty-five micrograms of the total cell lysate or 25 µl of the virus lysate containing 0.04% bromophenol blue were denatured at 95°C for 5 minutes and stored on ice for another 5 minutes. The denatured samples were separated by electrophoresis in a minigel containing 5% stacking and 8% resolving polyacrylamide gel containing SDS. The samples were first collected into the resolving gel phase at 80 volts per gel and then at 120 volts per gel once the samples entered the separating gel phase.

Western blotting of separated protein

The separated proteins were transferred onto nitrocellulose membrane at 0.8 mA/cm^2 for 1 hour (GE healthcare, Freiburg) using a 3-buffer semi-dry system as described below. The Whatmann paper and the nitrocellulose membrane were equilibrated in ethanol before they were wetted in their respective buffers. Three layers of Whatmann paper soaked in anode buffer I (300 mM Tris base, 20% v/v ethanol, pH 10.4) was placed on the positive plate of the blotting chamber, followed by another three layers of Whatmann paper saturated in buffer II (25 mM Tris base, 20% v/v ethanol, pH 10.4), and then by a layer of nitrocellulose membrane dampened in anode buffer II. Thereafter, the gel containing the separated proteins was transferred to the nitrocellulose membrane and was overlaid with three additional layers of Whatmann paper wetted in cathode buffer (25 mM Tris base, 20% v/v ethanol, 40 mM ε-aminocaproic acid, pH 9.4) before the sandwich was covered with the cathode plate. Once the blotting process was completed, the membrane was blocked with 5% (w/v) non-fat milk powder in PBS on a rocker for 1 hour. Blots were rinsed in PBST (PBS containing 0.01 % (v/v) Tween 20) and PVM protein were detected with 1:100 dilution of antiserum collected from rPVM-infected convalescent mice for 2 hours. The unbound antibiodies were removed with three changes of PBST for 5 minutes each and detected with goat-anti-mouse IgG coupled with HRP (1:2500) diluted in 5% (w/v) non-fat milk for 1 hour. The excess secondary antibodies were removed with three rounds of washing with PBST for 5 minutes each. The signal intensity of the stained membrane was developed with WesternBright™ chemiluminescence substrate (Biozym, Oldendorf) as described by the manufacturer. The images were recorded using the Fujifilm LAS 3000 CCD camera (Fujifilm, Dusseldorf) and quantified with the 2D-densiometry module of the AIDA software (v 3.20.116, Raytest Berlin).

2.2.10 Quantitative polymerase chain reaction (RT-qPCR)

RNA isolation and reverse transcription into cDNA

Total cellular RNA was collected from BHK-21 cells infected at MOI of 1 PFU/cell after 24 hours with the RNeasy RNA isolation kit (Qiagen) as specified by the manufacturer. One microgram of the RNA was treated with 1 unit of RNase free DNase I (Thermo-Scientific) for 30 minutes at 37°C to remove genomic DNA before the DNase was inactivated with 1 µl of 50 mm EDTA for 10 minutes at 65°C. The DNase-treated RNA was reverse transcribed as shown in section 2.2.5.

Real-time RCR assay

The synthesized cDNAs were diluted 1:10 with distilled water and quantified in triplicates using the iTaq universal SYBR Green supermix (Bio-Rad, Munich) and the primer pairs listed in table 8 on the ABI 7300 /7500 Real-Time PCR System (Applied Biosystems) using the conditions in table 9. The specificity and sizes of the PCR products were confirmed with the melt curve and gel electrophoresis (3% agarose gel), respectively.

Table 8: Primers for real time PCR (qPCR)

Forward primer	Reverse primer	Expected size (bp)
[a] PVM N Fw	[a] PVM N Rs	162
PVM G Fw	PVM G Rs	183
[a] PVM F Fw	[a] PVM F Rs	169
[b] 18s RNA Fw	[b]18s RNA Rs	140

Table 9: Reaction Setup for quantification of gene of interest by qPCR

<table>
<tr><td>Component</td><td>Volume</td><td colspan="2">Final concentration</td></tr>
<tr><td>iTaq Universal SYBR Green supermix (2X)</td><td>10 µl</td><td colspan="2">1 X</td></tr>
<tr><td>*Fw Primer (10 µM/ µl)</td><td>0.8 µl</td><td colspan="2">400 nM</td></tr>
<tr><td>*Rs Primer (10 µM/ µl)</td><td>0.8 µl</td><td colspan="2">400 nM</td></tr>
<tr><td>cDNA (diluted 1:10)</td><td>8 µl</td><td colspan="2"></td></tr>
<tr><td>H_2O</td><td>0.4 µl</td><td colspan="2"></td></tr>
<tr><td>Total reaction mix volume</td><td>20 µl</td><td colspan="2"></td></tr>
<tr><td>Program</td><td>Temperature</td><td>Time</td><td>Cycle</td></tr>
<tr><td>Activation of polymerase</td><td>95°C</td><td>10'</td><td>1 X</td></tr>
<tr><td>Denaturation</td><td>95°C</td><td>5''</td><td rowspan="2">40 X</td></tr>
<tr><td>Annealing and extension</td><td>60°C</td><td>1'</td></tr>
<tr><td>Melting curve: to confirm peak of products</td><td colspan="3">Default setting</td></tr>
</table>

* 18s rRNA primers were used at a final concentration of 300 nM.

The collected data were analysed using the LinRegPCR software (Ruijter et al., 2009). The N, F and G mRNA were first normalized to their respective 18s rRNA, then the normalized F and G mRNA were analysed relative to the normalized N mRNA.

2.2.11 Animal experiment

Intranasal infection of mice

Six to nine week-old mice were intranasally infected with a sublethal dose (150 PFU/80 µl of PBS) of virus suspension under 2 – 3 % isoflourane anaesthesia. Percentage weight gain or loss was determined relative to the initial weight just before infection was used to monitor virulence of the virus while clinical scores were based on conditions listed in table 10. Virus load in infected lungs at the amplification phase (day 3 postinfection) and at the peak of infection (day 6 postinfection) were determined as shown below.

Table 10: Clinical scores for animal experiment

Score	Symptoms
1	No symptoms
2	Roughened fur
3	Hunched posture, abnormal gait, difficulty breathing
4	Reduced mobility, cyanosis of ears and tail and lethargy (humane end Point)
5	Dead

Quantification of virus load in infected mouse lungs

Aseptically collected lung lobes were homogenized in 3 ml of complete EMEM medium supplemented with 10% (v/v) buffer containing 50 mM HEPES and 100 mM $MgSO_4$. The homogenates were clarified at 300 xg for 10 minutes at 4°C, aliquoted, frozen under nitrogen and stored at -80°C or used for virus load estimation by plaque assay as described in section 2.2.3.

2.2.12 Statistical analysis

Statistical analyses were performed with Prism 4.0 (GraphPad Inc, USA) and differences were considered significant if $p < 0.05$. All data were transformed with the common logarithm before use and assumed to be normally distributed. For kinetics studies where viruses were harvested every 24 hours, the overall median or mean difference between the tested groups was determined rather than differences at each time point as done for the experiments were viruses were collected at selected time points.

Groups of three were analysed using the one-way ANOVA followed by Dunnett's multiple comparison test if each time point was analysed or the repeated measures ANOVA followed by Bonferroni multiple comparison test if overall differences were tested. Groups of two were analysed with the paired T test if overall difference was determined while comparison at each time point was carried out using the unpaired T test with Welch's correction.

3. Results

3.1 PVM J3666 represents two distinct populations

Two variants of the PVM J3666-G gene have been described: (i) a variant containing two non-overlapping open reading frames (ORF) coding for a small uORF (uORF) that is potentially translated into a polypeptide of 12 amino acids and the main G ORF that encoded a G protein of 396 amino acids (Randhawa et al., 1995); (ii) in a second variant, the first uORF and the second ORF would be connected to form a single ORF that would be translated into a G protein of 414 amino acids due to the exchange of the stop codon of the uORF to a codon for lysine (Krempl and Collins, 2004). In the description of the second variant, the possibility of coexistence of both variants within the same virus preparation was suggested by the sequencing data of uncloned RT-PCR fragments. Due the time that has since elapsed, this latter observation was taken up and reinvestigated.

To determine the nucleotide (nt) composition of the G gene, BHK-21 cells were infected with a preparation of PVM J3666 that was successively derived from the stock used for the previous data. Total cellular RNA was collected, reverse transcribed with random hexamers and a fragment of 2,517 bp, herein referred to as J3666-MSHGF that covered 406 nucleotides of the M gene, the entire SH and G genes and 314 nucleotides in the F gene was amplified by PCR using a proofreading polymerase. The complete G gene of the uncloned fragment was sequenced and analysed with the SeqMan program (Lasergene v11, DNASTAR,).

Overlaying peaks were observed at nucleotide 65 that determine the presence of an uORF or the extension of the main ORF as described above (Figure 6A). Further polymorphisms were observed for nucleotides 104, 165 and 1121: positions 104 and 165 were within the putative portion of the gene coding for the cytoplasmic domain, while position 1121 was in the presumed ectodomain of the resulting protein (Figure 6B). Overlaying peaks for these positions had also been described earlier (Krempl and Collins, 2004). The polymorphisms at position 65 indicated an adenine (all nucleotides designations used refer to negative-stranded RNA sense) that would induce a stop codon or uracil that would lead to translation of lysine. If adenine was used, the first ORF initiating at AUG_{29} ended after 12 amino acids and the main G ORF would initiate at the downstream AUG_{83} coding for a G protein of 396 amino acids and enclosed a cytoplasmic domain of 35 amino acids. Whereas when lysine was encoded, the AUG_{29} and AUG_{83} were connected to a single G ORF that encoded a polypeptide of 414 amino acids (Figure 6A). The multiple peaks at nucleotide 104 represented by cytosine or uracil causing translation of glycine or serine, respectively; at nucleotide 165 was adenine or cytosine, inducing codons for valine, or glycine correspondingly; and at nucleotide 1121 was adenine for serine or uracil inducing the codon for threonine (Figure 6B). However, the consensus sequence contained uracil, cytosine, cytosine and uracil at nucleotides 65,104,165 and 1121, respectively, which would code for a G protein of 414 amino acids, although underlying peaks were quite prominent. Adenine as nucleotide 65, uracil as nucleotide 104, cytosine as nucleotide 165 and adenine as nucleotide 1121 corresponded to the G gene sequence published by Randhawa and colleagues (Randhawa et al., 1995) while uracil, cytosine, adenine and uracil at positions 65, 104, 165 and 1121, respectively, corresponded to the published G gene sequence of Krempl and Collins (Krempl and Collins, 2004). Thus, the determined consensus sequence represented a mixture of both published sequences. The results suggested that both G variants might coexist together within the analysed preparation of PVM J3666.

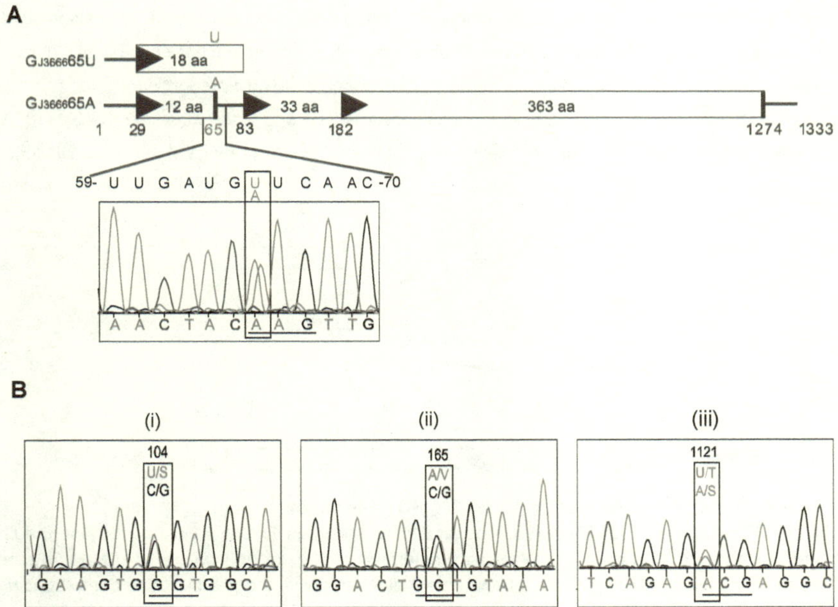

Figure 6: Analysis of the nucleotide composition of biological PVM strain J3666.
Total cellular RNA was subjected to RT-PCR using PVM-specific primer and the consensus sequence of the G gene was determined by direct sequencing of the amplified fragment. (A) Schematic representation of the G gene with consequent ORFs resulting from the nucleotide polymorphisms at position 65. ORFs are depicted as rectangles with potential start codons indicated by filled triangles and stop codons by a bar. The first and last nucleotides of the gene, and first nucleotides of translational start and stop codons are indicated. Below the drawing, a representative electropherogram of the sequencing reaction for position 59 to 70 of the G gene is shown. Note that sequence data are in positive sense, whereas the genomic sense RNA sequence is shown above. The overlaying peaks for nucleotide 65 representing the first nucleotide of the codon (underlined) for translational stop (TAG) and lysine (AAG), respectively, are boxed. (B) Representation of polymorphisms at positions 104 (i), 165 (ii), and 1121 (iii) found in the G gene: the specific nucleotide positions in the electropherogram are boxed. Sequence data are in positive sense and the corresponding codons are underlined. The nucleobases of genomic RNA (negative sense) and the resulting amino acid (single letter code) are shown above the electropherogram.

To determine the distribution of the observed polymorphisms within the PVM J3666 population, the amplified J3666-MSHGF fragments were cloned into plasmid vectors and 45 clones were sequenced. Out of the 45 clones analysed, 21 clones (47%) contained a G gene encoding a G ORF preceded by a separated uORF (nucleotide 65 A; $G_{J3666}65A$) and the remaining 24 clones (53%) would contain a single ORF coding for a N-terminally extended variant of the G protein (nucleotide 65 U; $G_{J3666}65U$) (Figure 7). Analysis of the clones with respect to the other variable positions revealed that all $G_{J3666}65A$-clones (n=21) encoded U at position 104 while all 17 $G_{J3666}65A$-clones analysed up to nucleotide 165 were found to encode C at that position. In addition, 5 of 6 randomly selected $G_{J3666}65A$-clones analysed until nucleotide 1121 were found to encode A at this position with the exception of one clone encoding U at this position. In comparison, the $G_{J3666}65U$-clones with a single exception encoded C at position 104 (23 of 24 clones), 20 out of 23 analysed up to nucleotide 165 contained U at that position and all four clones analysed at position 1121 encoded U. In summary, there appeared to be a predominantly homogeneous alignment of the nucleotide polymorphisms for positions 104, 165 and 1121 with either the $G_{J3666}65A$ or the $G_{J3666}65U$ form, thus indicating the possible coexistence of two discrete PVM J3666 populations.

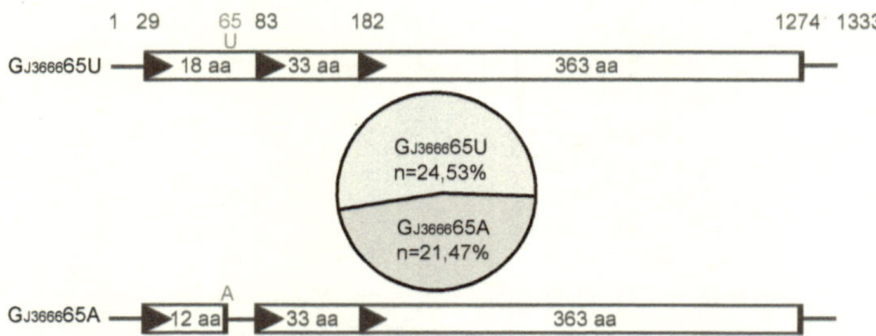

Figure 7: Clonal distribution of the PVM J3666-G gene variants.
The RT-PCR fragment (J3666-MSHGF) generated as shown in Figure 6 was cloned and the G-gene sequence of 45 individual clones was determined. The distribution of the J3666-G gene variants in the cloned J3666-MSHGF fragments is illustrated with the pie chart and corresponding ORFs resulting from the nucleotide polymorphisms at position 65 are shown below $G_{J3666}65A$ and above $G_{J3666}65U$. All indicated nucleotides represent negative sense RNA.

Table 11: Alignment of nucleotide polymorphisms for G-J3666 clones

G variants	Nucleotide position (rel. to G gene)			
	65	104	165	1121
$G_{J3666}65U$	U/Lys (24/24)	C/Gly (23/24) U/Ser (1/24)	A/Val (20/23) C/Gly (3/23)	U/Thr (4/4)
$G_{J3666}65A$	A/Stop (21/21)	U/Ser (21/21)	C/Gly (17/17)	A/Ser (5/6) U/Thr (1/6)

Nucleotides corresponding to the indicated positions within the G gene variants $G_{J3666}65U$ and $G_{J3666}65A$ (negative sense RNA) and the encoded amino acids are shown. The number of clones examined per location is indicated in the bracket: the numerator is the number of clones that contained the nucleobase shown in the table while the denominator is the total number of clones sampled per site of G gene variant.

To confirm this assumption, the sequence analysis was extended into the SH gene which has been reported to be polymorphic (Thorpe and Easton, 2005). The complete sequence of the SH gene of 40 out of the 45 clones analysed for G gene nucleotide composition were attainable and revealed 27 polymorphisms distributed throughout the gene that were majorly specific for either G_{J3666}65A- or G_{J3666}65U-clones. The SH gene of 16 of the 18 G_{J3666}65A-clones contained guanine at all the 27 positions while the remaining two clones contained adenine as found in the G_{J3666}65U-clones. All the 22 G_{J3666}65U-clones contained adenine at these polymorphic sites. The hypermutation affected the gene start, the ORF length and caused 17 amino acid substitutions between the SH variants (Figure 8). The polymorphisms at the positions 5 and 9 within the G_{J3666}65A-SH resulted in generation of a distinct gene start with no comparable sequence within the PVM genome. In addition, the G_{J3666}65A-SH mRNA would be translated into a polypeptide of 114 amino acids (stop codon position, nucleotides 353 – 355) while the G_{J3666}65U SH ORF consisted of 92 amino acids due to an early stop codon at nucleotides 287 – 289.

```
                                           H           P
GJ3666 65A UCCUGUUUGUUACCUAGGGUUGUACUGGAGUGUGGUCUAGUGGGGACUCUAGUUGUACUG 60
GJ3666 65U UCCUAUUUAUUACCUAGGAUUGUACUGGAGUAUGGUCUAGUGAAAACUCUAGUUGUACUG 60
                                           Y           F

                               H        P     P              P
GJ3666 65A GUCGUCGGCGUAACCGUGUGUGUAAUGUGGUCGGGGUUGUCGAGAAGAGGGACGUACACG 120
GJ3666 65U GUCGUCGGCAUAACCGUGUAUAUAAUGUGAUCGGGAUUGUCGAGAAGAGGAACGUACACG 120
                               Y        L     L              L

                         A  R                 R
GJ3666 65A GCAGUAGUUGUGUCGCGCACGCGACUAUUACCGGGCGUCGUCAUCUUCGUAGCGAUGUAG 180
GJ3666 65U GCAGUAGUUGUGUCACACACGCGACUAUUACCGGACGUCGUCAUCUUCGUAACGAUGUAG 180
                         V  C                 C

                              R                                H
GJ3666 65A UCCGUAACAGUCGUCGGUUGCGUGUCAAGUAGGGUUAGUGGGAGGUGGUUCAGUACCGCA 240
GJ3666 65U UCCGUAACAGUCGUCGGUUACGUGUCAAGUAGGGUUAGUGGGAGGUGGUUCAAUACCGCA 240
                              C                                Y

                A                    P H                   Q    H    Q
GJ3666 65A GUUACGUUGACCAGACGGCCCAUUGGGUGUGAGUUCCUUGUGGUGUGUUGUGGUAUUUGU 300
GJ3666 65U GUUACAUUGACCAGACGGCCCAUUGGAUAUGAGUUCCUUGUGAUGUAUUGUAAUAUUUAU 300
                V                    L Y

GJ3666 65A UGUCUUUAAUAGGAAGUUAUUUGGGUCCGGUCUGUCGAAAUGGACGAUCUACUAAGUU 360
GJ3666 65U UGUCUUUAAUAGGAAGUUAUUUGGGUCCGGUCUGUCGAAAUGGACGAUCUACUAAGUU 360

GJ3666 65A AGUCGGAAACGUCAUACAGCAGAUCAAUUGUUUUUU 396
GJ3666 65U AGUCGGAAACGUCAUACAGCAGAUCAAUUGUUUUUU 396
```

Figure 8: Alignment of the SH genes of G_{J3666}65A and G_{J3666}65U.
The consensus sequences of the G_{J3666}65A SH (16 clones) and G_{J3666}65U SH (22 clones) were derived from the alignment of their respective clones. The gene start signal is underlined, the 27 nucleotides differences are shaded and the nonsynonymous amino acid changes are shown above, and below their codons with a single-letter code. The stop codons of the 92 amino acids SH ORF and the 114 amino acids SH ORF are boxed. All indicated sequences are shown for the negative-stranded RNA.

The primers used for the analysis of the SH gene covered 50 terminal nucleotides of the M gene of 36 J3666-MSHGF clones. Therefore, this portion was also analysed. The analysis of this portion revealed that the purine hypermutation observed in the SH gene continued into the M gene: 12 of 16 of the G_{J3666}65A clones contained guanine at 7 polymorphic positions, 2 contained guanine at 6 of the 7 polymorphic sites and the sequences of 2 clones were not obtainable. Thus, the 12 clones described above contained guanine at all polymorphic sites within the M and SH genes. The M genes of the G_{J3666}65U clones (19 out of 20) contained adenine at all 7 polymorphic positions with the exception of one clone that contained guanine (Figure 9). Of note, three of the polymorphic sites were within the gene end signal of the M gene (nucleotides 922, 923 and 927) to produce a distinct gene end for the M genes of the G_{J3666}65A clones.

```
nt position 895                                   931
                            T     T
GJ3666 65A M    GGUGUGUGUAUAUGUGUGUGUAGGAUCGGUUUGUUUU
GJ3666 65U M    GGUGUAUGUAUAUAUGUGUAUAGAAUCAAUUUAUUUU
                            I     I
```

Figure 9: Alignment of the M genes of G_{J3666}65A and G_{J3666}65U.
The consensus sequences of the M genes of the G_{J3666}65A and G_{J3666}65U clones were derived from the alignment of the respective sequence data. The gene end signals of the M genes are underlined and the stop codons are boxed. The nucleotide differences are shaded while the predicted amino acids are indicated with single-letter code. All indicated sequences are shown for negative-stranded RNA.

In conclusion, because the majority of the clones examined could be separated into two distinct populations with respect to the sequence of their M, SH and G genes, the analysed quasispecies of PVM J3666 was considered to represent two discrete populations. In consequence, the virus stock was renamed PVM J3666 (G_{J3666}65AU) to reflect its constituents.

3.2 Contribution of the PVM-G gene organisation to replication and virulence

To evaluate and characterize the different G genes found in the quasispecies of PVM J3666 relative to the G gene found in PVM 15, a reverse genetics approach was used to generate PVM mutants differing exclusively in their G genes (Figure 10). The system for generating recombinant PVM (rPVM) is based on PVM 15, thus the recombinant wild-type virus and parent for the mutants contains a G gene encoding a G protein of 396 amino acids similar to G_{J3666}65A but without the uORF (Krempl et al., 2007). The newly generated viruses were: rPVM-G_{J3666}65A and rPVM-G_{J3666}65U that contained the variants of the PVM J3666-G gene in place of the PVM 15-G gene. This approach allowed the direct comparison of the effects of the extension of the main G ORF and the presence of an uORF, respectively, on the synthesis of the G protein and on replication and virulence of the viruses.

3.2.1 Generation of recombinant PVM containing the G_{J3666}65A and G_{J3666}65U

rPVM was recovered from pPVM, a plasmid containing the full-length antigenomic cDNA of PVM 15 under the control of the promoter of the T7 polymerase. Briefly, using a subgenomic plasmid containing the complete G, F and M2 genes of PVM 15, the variant defining region of the G gene was substituted for that of G_{J3666}65A or G_{J3666}65U, respectively. PCR fragments encompassing G_{J3666}65A or G_{J3666}65U, respectively, were amplified from confirmed clones of J3666-MSHGF using a forward primer that added an *Age*I restriction site immediately upstream of the G gene start signal and an antisense primer that bound in the F gene. Of note, the *Age*I site is unique for the rPVM genome and does not occur in biological derived PVM. A fragment encompassing nucleotide 1 to 931 of the PVM 15-G gene was replaced with the corresponding G_{J3666}65U-PCR fragment using unique *Age*I and *Avr*II restriction sites (positions 4510 and 5441 relative to rPVM genome) as shown in Figure 10. Thus, the resulting chimeric G gene also contained the nucleotide substitutions at nucleotide 104, 165 and 1121 specific for the G_{J3666}65U population since the latter nucleotides are identical between strain 15 and J3666 65U.

For generation of G_{J3666}65A, an *Age*I site was added accordingly and a fragment containing the complete G gene and 155 nucleotide of the adjacent F gene up to a unique *Nde*I restriction site (position 6020 relative to the rPVM genome) was substituted for that of the G_{J3666}65A subpopulation. The sequence of the G-F intergenic region and the first 155 nucleotides of the F gene are similar between strains 15 and J3666 for the. Thus, despite the differing cloning strategies, the resulting rPVM mutants differed exclusively in their G genes with the complete respective G gene equalling that of the J3666 subpopulations. After confirmation of the resulting subclones by sequencing, the GFM2 fragment of pPVM was exchanged for the respective G_{J3666}FM2 fragments. The integrity of the selected full-length plasmids pPVM-G_{J3666}65A and pPVM-G_{J3666}65U was confirmed by restriction endonuclease digestion with *Acc*I, *Hind*III, *Nde*I and *Pac*I as reported in Figure 11.

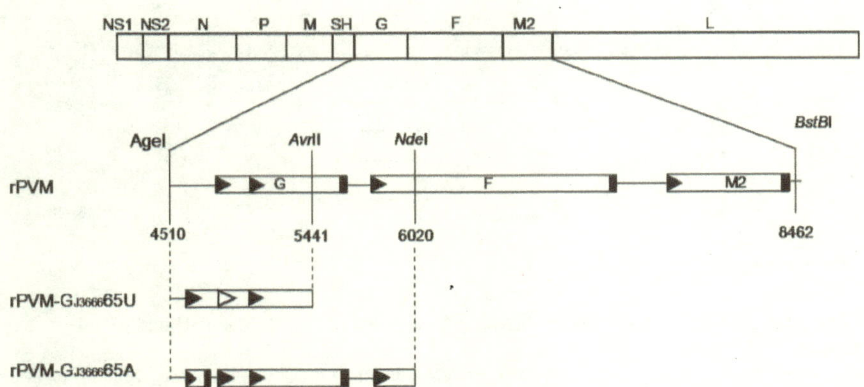

Figure 10: Schematic representation of the generation of rPVM encoding the two distinct J3666-G gene variants.

All changes were performed using a plasmid containing an antigenomic cDNA fragment encoding the G, F and M2 genes flanked by unique *AgeI* and *BstBI* restriction enzyme sites for reassembly of the antigenomic full-length plasmid (Krempl et al., 2007). Fragments of J3666 G containing the 65U or 65A nucleotide, respectively, as well as other variant determining nucleotides were amplified from plasmids using a forward primer adding the *AgeI* restriction site that is specific for recombinant PVM (Krempl et al., 2007). The original G strain 15 fragment as indicated in the drawing was exchanged with the corresponding fragments specific of G_{J3666}65U and G_{J3666}65A. Nucleotide sequences between position 4510 and 6020 of the genomic sequence were confirmed by sequencing. Nucleotide positions of restriction enzyme sites are given relative to the rPVM genome.

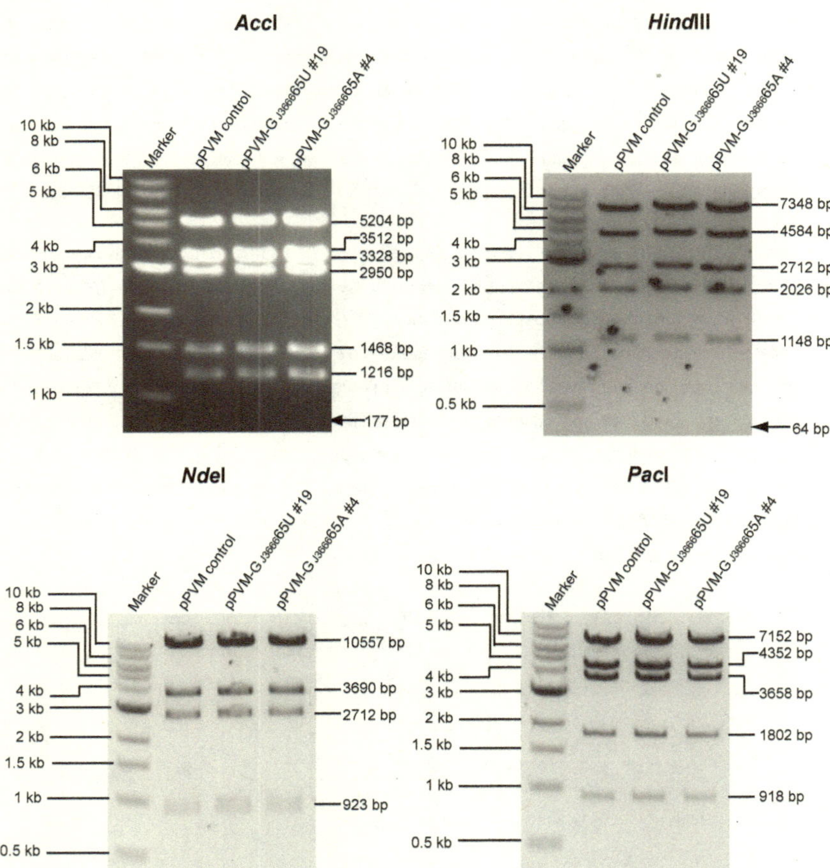

Figure 11: Diagnostic restriction of full-length plasmids of pPVM-G$_{J3666}$65U and pPVM-G$_{J3666}$65A.

Full-length clones used for isolation of the rPVM variants, i.e. pPVM-G$_{J3666}$65A clone 4, pPVM-G$_{J3666}$65U clone 19, and pPVM as control, were digested with *Acc*I, *Hind*III, *Nde*I or *Pac*I, respectively. The digested samples were resolved by agarose gel electrophoresis and the resulting bands were compared to those of pPVM. The fragment sizes of the DNA marker (1 kb ladder, NEB) are indicated on the left side of the images while the expected sizes of the plasmid fragments are on the right side. Note that fragment sizes of pPVM-G$_{J3666}$65A and pPVM-G$_{J3666}$65U are expected to be identical to those of pPVM.

rPVM-G$_{J3666}$65U and rPVM-G$_{J3666}$65A were isolated by transfecting BSR-T7/5 cells that constitutively express the T7 RNA polymerase, with the selected full-length plasmids together with a cocktail of plasmids expressing the subunits of the PVM polymerase (N, P, M2-1 and L proteins) also under the control of the T7 promoter (see section 2.2.8). The recovered viruses were propagated in BHK-21 cells and at the third passage both recombinant virus preparations had reached titres of more than 10^6 PFU/ml (Table 12). The nucleotide sequence of the G genes of the rPVM mutants was confirmed by direct sequencing of RT-PCR fragments produced from total cellular RNA collected from infected BHK-

21 cells after the third passage. All following infection experiments were performed using these confirmed virus preparations.

Table 12: Titre development of the newly isolated rPVM-G variants over the first three passages

Virus	Passage 1	Passage 2	Passage 3
rPVM-G_{J3666}65A	3.07 x 10^4 PFU/ml	9.3 x 10^5 PFU/ml	6.9 x 10^6 PFU/ml
rPVM-G_{J3666}65U	5.3 x 10^3 PFU/ml	3.7 x 10^6 PFU/ml	5.07 x 10^6 PFU/ml

3.2.2 The G gene organization affected the expression level of the G protein

First, the effect of the uORF preceding the main G ORF in rPVM-G_{J3666}65A and of the possible extension of the main ORF in rPVM-G_{J3666}65U on the expression of the G protein was investigated by Western blot analysis of BHK-21 cell lysates collected after infection for 4 days with rPVM or rPVM-G_{J3666}65A or rPVM-G_{J3666}65U, respectively. Protein levels were quantified by chemiluminescence imaging using the LAS 3000 CCD camera (Fujifilm, Düsseldorf) and the AIDA software (v 3.20.116, Raytest Berlin). The G protein levels were analysed relative to that of the intrinsic P protein for each virus.

The normalization of the G protein signal intensity to the signal intensity of the P protein indicated that the presence of the uORF preceding the main G ORF in the G_{J3666}65A gene reduced G protein expression by 1.8-fold compared to the expression of the G protein in rPVM-infected cells (Figure 12A and B). In comparison, the extension of the G ORF in the corresponding gene of rPVM-G_{J3666}65U rather caused a 1.5-fold increase in the amount of G protein produced in infected cells relative to G protein levels in rPVM-infected cells. The G protein expression in rPVM-G_{J3666}65U infected cells increased by 2.5-fold compared to rPVM-G_{J3666}65A-infected cells (Figure 12B).

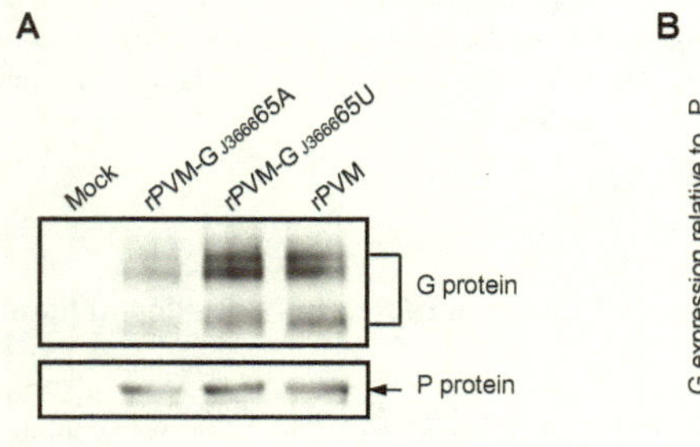

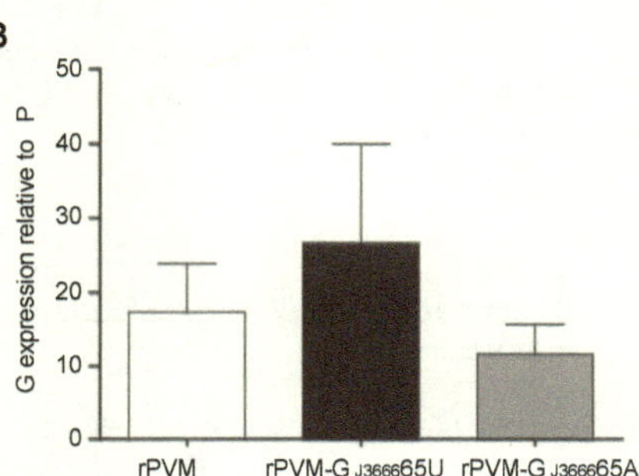

Figure 12: G protein expression by the rPVM-G gene variants.
(A) The expression of G protein was determined in cell lysates collected from BHK-21 cells infected with rPVM, rPVM-G_{J3666}65A or rPVM-G_{J3666}65U, respectively, at a multiplicity of infection (MOI) of 0.1 PFU/cell for 4 days by Western blotting. Proteins were detected by immunostaining using serum from convalescent mice infected with rPVM, combined with chemiluminescence imaging using the LAS 3000 CCD camera (Fujifilm). (B) Blots from two independent experiments as exemplified in A,

were quantified using the AIDA software (v 3.20.116, Raytest Berlin). For each lane, the signals of the G bands per lane were normalized to the P signal. Bars represent the standard errors between the runs.

To exclude any transcriptional effect on the observed differences in G protein expression, the G mRNA levels were determined by quantitative RT-PCR. Since the transcription of genes occurs sequentially, two other genes, N and F, were selected alongside the G gene to deduce the events upstream and downstream of the gene. Each mRNA level was normalized to the 18s rRNA and then expressed as the ratio of the N mRNA for each virus (Figure 13). The analysis revealed that the selected genes were transcribed at similar rates and the levels of G mRNAs (0.9-fold to 1.5-fold over N) varied somewhat more than those of F mRNAs (0.64-fold to 0.69-fold over N). Consequently, the differences in the G protein expression noted for the three rPVMs were independent of transcription. Thus, it appeared that the uORF reduced the translation of the downstream G ORF while the extension of the ORF favoured increased G protein expression.

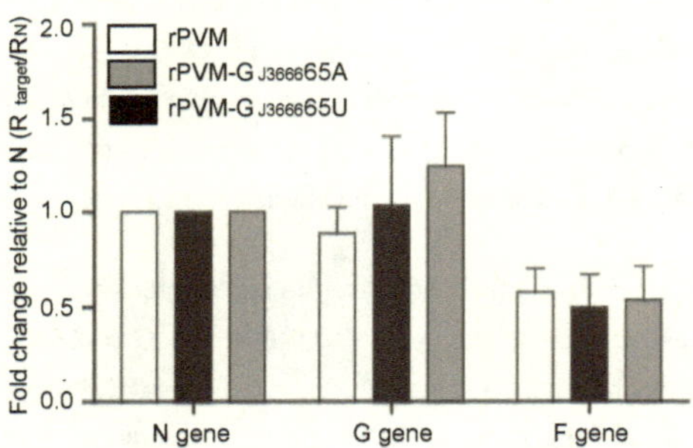

Figure 13: Transcription of N, G and F genes in cells infected with the rPVM-G gene variants
The transcription rate of the G, F and N genes was determined by SYBR green-based qRT-PCR. Total cellular RNA was isolated from BHK-21 cells infected as described for Figure 6, reverse transcribed with random hexamers and subjected to qPCR with primers specific for the indicated genes. The data were analysed with the LinRegPCR program (Ruijter et al., 2009). The result for each target gene was normalized to 18s rRNA and expressed as fold change relative to the amount of N mRNA. Error bars represent the standard deviation between two independent runs each performed in triplicates.

3.2.3 Effects of the J3666-G gene variants on multicycle replication kinetics in tissue culture

The effect of the G_{J3666} variants on PVM replication in BHK-21 cells and RAW 264.7 cells was compared to that of the parental rPVM following an infection with a multiplicity of infection (MOI) of 0.01 PFU/cell. Cell monolayers were infected in duplicates, and cells and medium supernatants were collected on days 1, 3, 5 and 7 postinfection. Cell-bound viruses were released by three freeze-thaw cycles, followed by centrifugation to collect the supernatants that were flash-frozen and stored until titrated on Vero cells by plaque assay.

In BHK-21 cells, rPVM-G_{J3666}65A and rPVM appeared to replicate equally at day 1 to reach a mean titre of 1.6 x 10^2 PFU/ml and 1.5 x 10^2 PFU/ml, respectively. By day 3 postinfection, rPVM-G_{J3666}65A outgrew rPVM by 3-fold to reach a mean titre of 2.6 x 10^4 PFU/ml compared to a mean titre of 8.6 x 10^3 PFU/ml for rPVM. On day 5 postinfection, the average titre of rPVM-G_{J3666}65A (3.3 x 10^5 PFU/ml) was 4-fold higher than the mean titre of 8.1 x 10^4 PFU/ml recorded for rPVM. By day 7, the mean titre of rPVM-G_{J3666}65A at 4.08 x 10^6 PFU/ml was approximately 6-fold higher than that of rPVM at 6.7 x 10^5 PFU/ml. In comparison, the replication patterns of rPVM-G_{J3666}65U and rPVM were comparable at all four time-points (Figure 14A). Therefore, the presence of an uORF in the G gene of rPVM-G_{J3666}65A appeared to enhance its replication in BHK-21 cells despite the reductive effect on the expression of the G protein, while the increased production of the G protein by rPVM-G_{J3666}65U appeared not to contribute to replication. The overall difference between the virus titres of rPVM and rPVM-G_{J3666}65A was statistically significant ($p < 0.05$).

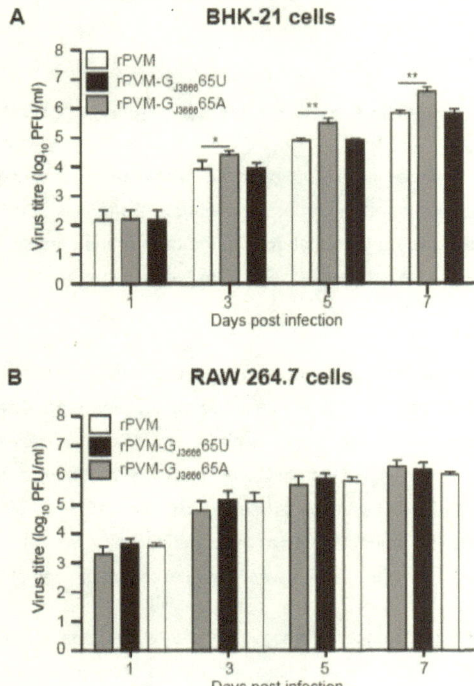

Figure 14: The G_{J3666}65A variant encoding an uORF promotes replication in BHK-21 but not in RAW 264.7

BHK-21 or RAW 264.7 cells were infected with rPVM, rPVM-G_{J3666}65U or rPVM-G_{J3666}65A at an MOI of 0.01 PFU/cell. At the indicated time points, cells and supernatants were harvested, subjected to freeze-thaw cycles to detach cell-bound virus particles, clarified from debris and stored for determination of virus titre by plaque assay. Data points represent mean values of two independent experiments performed in duplicates. Standard error is represented by error bar. Statistical analysis was carried out using one-way ANOVA test followed by Dunnett's multiple comparison test; rPVM-

$G_{J366665}$A and rPVM-$G_{J366665}$U were compared to rPVM as the control. Differences were considered significant at $p < 0.05$.

In contrast, in the murine RAW 264.7 cells, rPVM-$G_{J366665}$A, rPVM-$G_{J366665}$U and rPVM replicated with comparable kinetics at all-time points investigated (Figure 14B). On days 1, 3 and 5 postinfection, rPVM and rPVM-$G_{J366665}$U replicated about 2-fold higher than rPVM-$G_{J366665}$A. By day 7, rPVM-$G_{J366665}$A mean titre was 1.9 x 10^6 PFU/ml compared to 1.5 x 10^6 PFU/ml and 1.1 X 10^6 PFU/ml recorded for rPVM-$G_{J366665}$U and rPVM, respectively. There was however no overall statistical difference between the growth kinetics of the viruses ($p > 0.05$). These results indicated that the different G gene variants were capable of supporting the replication of the respective virus at equal rate in RAW 264.7 cells.

In conclusion, the downregulation of G protein levels by the presence of an uORF indicated a slight advantage for replication of PVM in a cell line-specific fashion whereas the extension of the G ORF or upregulation of the G protein did not affect the replication efficiency.

3.2.4 The composition of the G gene affects the virulence of PVM in BALB/c mice

Lastly, the effect of the differences in composition of the PVM-G genes on virulence and replication was investigated by infecting BALB/c mice intranasally with 150 PFU/mouse of rPVM-$G_{J366665}$A or rPVM-$G_{J366665}$U or rPVM, representing a sublethal dose in the case of the parental virus. The body weight was daily recorded and disease was expressed as the percentage weight loss relative to the initial weight at day 0.

Symptomatic disease exemplified by ruffled fur and reduced activity (data not shown) was observed from day 8 until day 12 postinfection and all mice subsequently recovered. Disease severity was most prominent in rPVM-$G_{J366665}$U-infected mice, declining in rPVM-infected mice and was almost asymptomatic following infection with rPVM-$G_{J366665}$A. The highest difference in weight loss was at day 9 postinfection when rPVM-$G_{J366665}$U-infected mice had lost about 10% of their initial weight compared to 6% weight loss documented for rPVM-infected mice and about 1% weight loss for rPVM-$G_{J366665}$A-infected mice (Figure 15A). However, all mice were convalescent at the end of the experiment.

To determine if the observed difference in pathogenicity of the PVM variants in BALB/c mice was based on different replication efficiencies, the virus load in the lungs of the infected mice was determined at days 3 and 6 postinfection, which represent the amplification phase and the peak of virus replication, respectively. The lungs were removed from infected mice at these days, homogenized, and used for determination of the virus load by plaque assay. At day 3 postinfection, the average virus load of 7.5 x 10^2 PFU/lung in rPVM-$G_{J366665}$A-infected mice was comparable to mean titre of 5.8 x 10^2 PFU/lung from mice infected with rPVM. However, the mean titre in lungs of rPVM-$G_{J366665}$U-infected mice was 1.4 x 10^3 PFU/lung (Figure 15B). At day 6 postinfection, the mean virus load in the lungs of all infected mice was comparable. rPVM-$G_{J366665}$U-infected mice had a mean pulmonary titre of 5.5 x 10^5 PFU/lung, the mean virus load of rPVM-$G_{J366665}$A-infected mouse lungs was 3.7 x 10^5 PFU/lung and the lungs of rPVM-infected mice also had a mean titre of 3.8 x 10^5 PFU/lung (Figure 15b). The results showed that rPVM-G$_{J3666}$65U, rPVM-G$_{J3666}$65A and rPVM replicated efficiently in the lungs of infected animal but with varying levels of virulence.

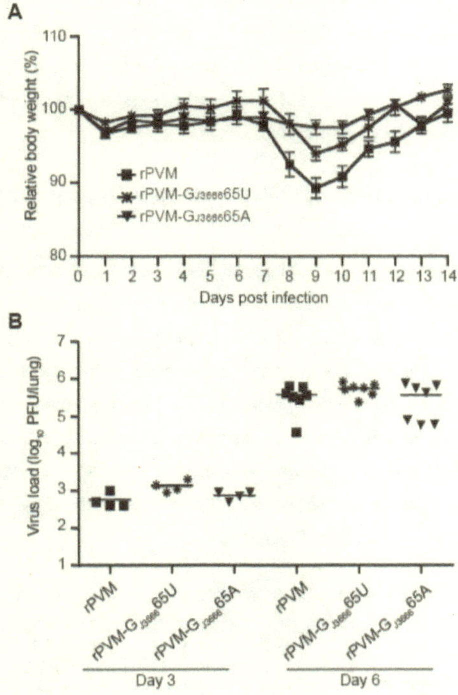

Figure 15: Replication and virulence of rPVM varying in the organization of G genes in mice.

BALB/c mice were intranasally infected with 150 PFU of the indicated viruses. (A) For comparison of virulence, mice in groups of 5 were infected intranasally with rPVM-G$_{J3666}$65A or rPVM-G$_{J3666}$65U, respectively, whereas 4 mice were infected with rPVM. Mice were weighed daily and closely observed for clinical scores. (B) For determination of the virus load, mice were infected as described for A, 4 mice and 7 mice per group were sacrificed at days 3 and 6 postinfection, respectively. The lungs were removed, homogenized and virus titres were determined by plaque assay.

3.3 The G gene determines the replication phenotype of biological PVM strains

The analysis of the rPVM-G gene variants demonstrated that the structure of the G gene affected G protein levels and replication efficiency in a particular cell line. However, compared to the rPVM-G gene variants, the biological PVM strains including the two PVM J3666 populations differed in additional genetic features such as the SH and M genes (see section 3.1 and chapter 1). Therefore, experiments in this section were designed to determine if the specific G gene variations are also reflected in the phenotype of their biological PVM strain parents.

3.3.1 Selection of individual PVM-J3666 populations by sequential passaging in tissue culture

Since the G gene variants present in the PVM J3666 (G_{J3666}65AU) had different properties with respect to the level of G protein expression and the replication kinetics in BHK-21 cells, the mixed stock containing the two populations was sequentially passaged in BHK-21 cells to evaluate if any of these differing properties of the G genes would confer a selective advantage to one of the populations. Following each passage, total cellular RNA was collected from infected BHK-21 cells and used to produce J3666-MSHGF fragment as described in section 3.1. Thereafter, portion of the G gene covering the first 165 nucleotides of the G gene was sequenced. After seven passages in BHK-21 cells, homogenous peaks were observed for positions 65, 104 and 165 of the G gene, indicating that a single population of the virus had been selected (Figure 16).

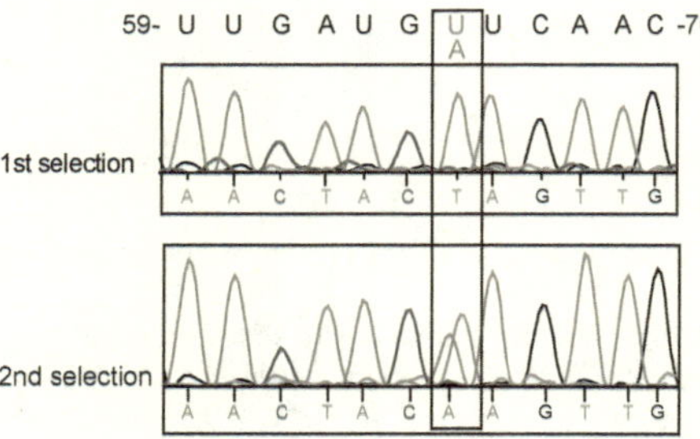

Figure 16: Sequential passage in BHK-21 cells appears to favour the G gene version containing an uORF.
Sequence analysis of the G gene of PVM J3666 after two separate selection experiments in BHK-21 cells. After the final round of selection, total cellular RNA was isolated from infected cells, the J3666-MSHGF fragment was amplified by sequence-specific RT-PCR and the G genes were sequenced directly. Shown are the electropherograms from positions 59 to 70 of the G genes after 7 (1st experiment, top panel) and 8 passages (2nd experiment, bottom panel), respectively. Peaks for nucleotide 65 representing the first nucleotide of the anticodon for translational stop (AUC) or lysine (UUC) are boxed. Indicated nucleotides are for negative sense RNA whereas sequence data are in positive sense.

Subsequently, the J3666-MSHGF fragment was cloned into a plasmid vector and 13 individual clones were selected and sequenced in their entirety. The sequence analysis of the complete J3666-MSHGF insert confirmed that a single virus population consisting entirely of the G_{J3666}65A variant had been selected as the M and SH genes were also similar to the M and SH genes identified when the mixed stock was resolved by cloning (section 3.1.2). In addition, a substitution at nucleotide 416 of the G gene (cytosine to uracil) leading to translation of glycine instead of threonine (T112G) was identified in all clones that was not present in the G_{J3666}65A population prior to the sequential passage. However, the selection of a single population was not reproducible when repeated in either BHK-21 cells or RAW 264.7 cells (not shown), indicating that each variant is capable of efficient replication in cell culture and that the mixed populations probably did not result from adaptation processes in tissue culture. The isolated virus variant was named PVM J3666 (G_{J3666}65A) and was propagated once more in BHK-21 cells to produce virus stock for later studies.

3.3.2 The level of G protein synthesis differs between biological PVM isolates

It was hypothesized that the expression of G protein by the biological strains would be similar to observations made with the recombinant viruses. To test this hypothesis, the amount viral proteins in BHK-21 cell lysates collected after 4 days of infection at MOI = 0.1 PFU/cell was analysed by Western blotting and the protein levels were quantified as described in 3.2.2.

The amount of G protein produced in infected cells was in the order PVM 15 > PVM J3666 (G_{J3666}65AU) > PVM J3666 (G_{J3666}65A) (Figure 17A). Normalization of the signal intensity of the G glycoprotein to that of the P protein indicated that G expression was 1.2-fold higher in cells infected with PVM 15 than in cells infected with PVM J3666 (G_{J3666}65AU), and 1.8-fold higher than in cells infected with PVM J3666 (G_{J3666}65A) indicating that the G protein expression is repressed by the uORF in the PVM J3666 G gene (Figure 17B). G protein expression in cells infected with PVM J3666 (G_{J3666}65AU) was 1.2-fold higher than in cells infected with PVM J3666 (G_{J3666}65A).

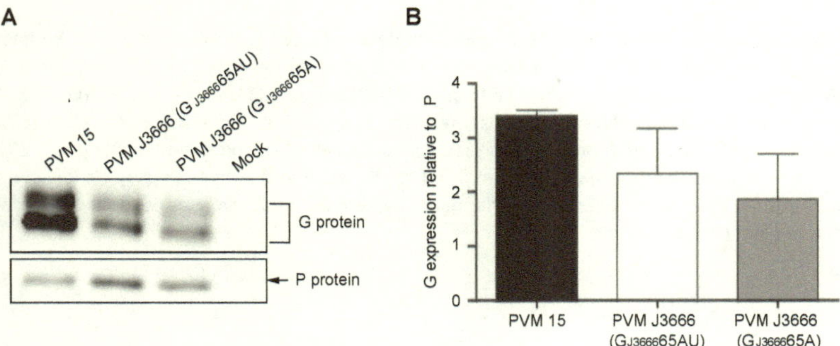

Figure 19: Analysis of G protein expression in BHK-21 cells infected with biological PVM isolates.

(A) BHK-21 cells, mock infected or infected with the indicated PVM strains, were lysed at day 4 postinfection and subjected to Western blot analysis. PVM proteins were detected with serum from rPVM-infected convalescent mice combined with chemiluminescence imaging. (B) Blots from two independent infections were quantified using the AIDA software (v 3.20.116, Raytest Berlin). For each lane, the signals of the G protein per lane were normalized to the signal of the P protein. Error bars represent the standard error between the runs.

Next, it was important to determine if the observed differences in G protein levels between the biological isolates were due to variation in their transcription pattern. Therefore, total-cellular RNA from BHK-21 cells infected with PVM J3666 (G_{J3666}65A) or PVM 15 or PVM J3666 (G_{J3666}65AU) at MOI of 1 PFU/cell were collected for mRNA quantification by qRT-PCR. Since the transcription of genes occurs sequentially, two other genes, N and F, were selected alongside the G gene so that events upstream and downstream of the gene could also be assessed. Each viral mRNA was first normalized to the respective 18s rRNA and later expressed as a ratio of the normalized N mRNA levels. The transcription rate of the G and F mRNAs within the mixed genomes of PVM J3666 (G_{J3666}65AU) was comparable to that of the homogenous genomes of PVM J3666 (G_{J3666}65A) and PVM 15 (Figure 18). Thus, reaffirming that the effect of the G gene organization on the translation of the G glycoprotein by the biological isolates. In conclusion, the difference in G protein levels among the biological isolates was independent of transcription as previously reported for the recombinant viruses.

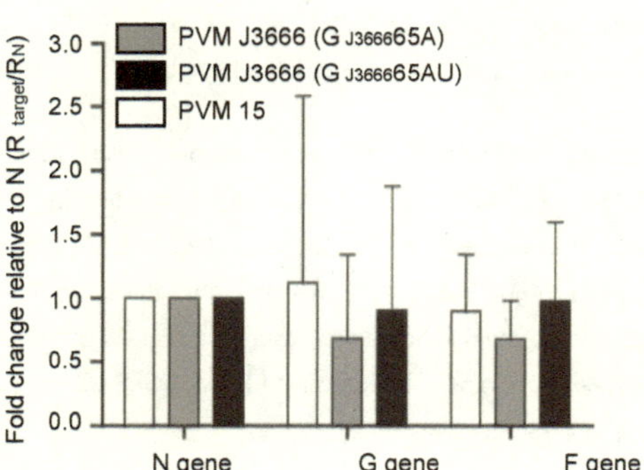

Figure 18: Transcription of N, G, and F genes in cells infected with biological PVM isolates. The transcription rate of virus genes was determined by SYBR green based qRT-PCR. Total cellular RNA from BHK-21 cells infected with PVM15 or PVM J3666 (G_{J3666}65A) or PVM J3666 (G_{J3666}65AU) were reverse transcribed with random hexamers and subjected to qPCR with primers specific for the indicated mRNAs. The data were analysed with the LinRegPCR program (Ruijter et al., 2009). Target mRNA in each group was first normalized to 18s rRNA and then expressed as fold change over N mRNA. Error bars represent the standard deviation between two independent experiments performed in triplicates.

3.3.3 The biological PVM isolates exhibit different replication kinetics in tissue culture

The replication efficiency of PVM J3666 (G_{J3666}65A) and PVM J3666 (G_{J3666}65AU) against the reference strain PVM 15 was evaluated in tissue culture. BHK-21 or RAW 264.7 cells were infected with the biological PVM isolates at an MOI of 0.01 PFU/cell. At the indicated time points, cells and supernatants were harvested from infected-BHK-21 cells while only supernatants were collected from infected-RAW 264.7 cells. Virus titres were determined by plaque assay on Vero cells.

In BHK-21 cells, the mean titre of PVM J3666 (G_{J3666}65AU) at 3.3 x 10^3 PFU/ml on day 1 postinfection was 12-fold and 8-fold higher than that of PVM 15 (2.7 x 10^2 PFU/ml) and PVM J3666 (G_{J3666}65A) (4.1 x 10^2 PFU/ml), respectively, (Figure 19A). This trend continued until day 3, when the differences started to level off. The mean titre of 2.4 x 10^5 PFU/ml for PVM J3666 (G_{J3666}65AU) was only 2-fold higher than that of PVM J3666 (G_{J3666}65A) at 9.4 x 10^4 PFU/ml and 6-fold more than the titre of PVM 15 at 4.1 x 10^4 PFU/ml.

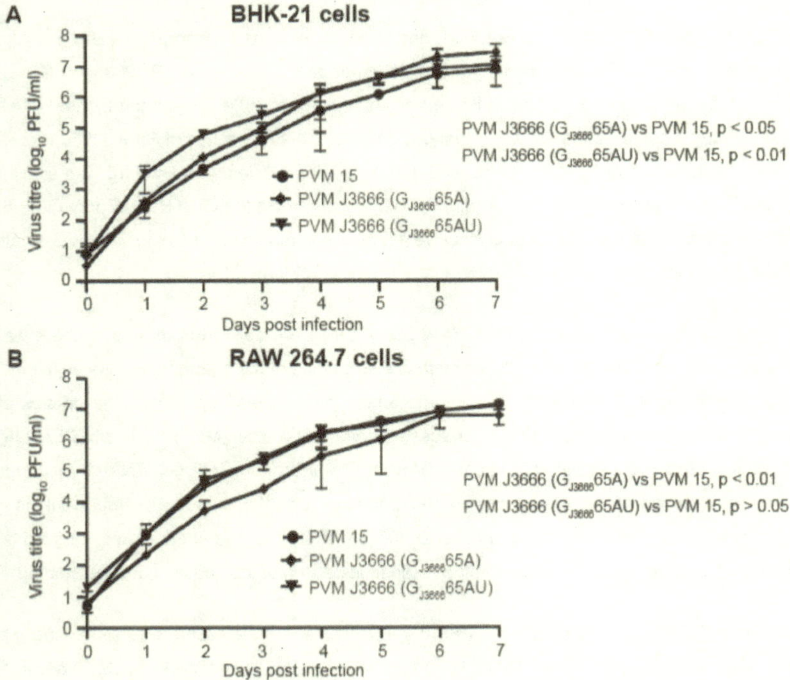

Figure 19: The replication of PVM J3666 (G_{J3666}65A) is attenuated in RAW 264.7 cells but not in BHK-21 cells.

Multi-cycle replication kinetics of PVM 15, PVM J3666 (G_{J3666}65A) and PVM J3666 (G_{J3666}65AU) in BHK-21 cells (A) and RAW 264.7 cells (B). Cells were infected at an MOI of 0.01 PFU/cell, and at the indicated time points, cells and supernatants were harvested for BHK-21 and supernatants were collected from infected RAW 264.7 cells. Titres were determined by plaques assay on Vero cells under methylcellulose. Each data point represents the mean value of two independent experiments performed in duplicates. Error bars indicate the standard deviation between runs. Repeated measures ANOVA followed by Bonferroni multiple comparison test were used to compare PVM J3666 (G_{J3666}65A) and PVM J3666 (G_{J3666}65AU) to PVM 15. Differences were considered significant at $p < 0.05$.

By days 4 and 5 postinfection, PVM J3666 (G_{J3666}65AU) and PVM J3666 (G_{J3666}65A) had comparable replication pattern with mean titres of about 4 x 10^6 PFU/ml on day 5 against a mean titre of 2 x 10^6 PFU/ml recorded for PVM 15. On day 6, the mean titre of PVM 15 (6 x 10^6 PFU/ml) was similar to the mean titre of PVM J3666 (G_{J3666}65AU) (8 x 10^6 PFU/ml), but was about 3-fold lower than the mean titre of PVM J3666 (G_{J3666}65A) at 2 x 10^7 PFU/ml. On day 7, the mean titre of PVM 15 at 8 x 10^6 PFU/ml was 3.5-fold and 1.7-fold lower than that of PVM J3666 (G_{J3666}65A) at 2.8 x 10^7 PFU/ml and PVM J3666 (G_{J3666}65AU) at 1.3 x 10^7 PFU/ml, respectively. Overall, the mixed PVM J3666 isolate replicated faster at the beginning of the time course with the differences levelling off at later time points, whereas the homogenous PVM J3666 isolate had a replication advantage at later time points, thus, rather behaving comparable to the corresponding rPVM-G_{J3666}65A. The PVM 15 replication efficiency was lower than that of PVM J3666 (G_{J3666}65A) ($p <0.05$) and PVM J3666 (G_{J3666}65AU) ($p <0.01$).

In RAW 264.7 cells, PVM J3666 (G_{J3666}65AU) and PVM 15 replicated similarly from day 1 until day 7 postinfection to reach mean titres of 1.2 X 10^7 PFU/ml at day 7. In contrast, PVM J3666 (G_{J3666}65A) appeared moderately attenuated for the first 4 days compared to PVM 15 with the highest difference occurring on day 3 postinfection (8-fold). From day 5 onward, the replication of PVM J3666 (G_{J3666}65A) was comparable to that of PVM 15. In general, the replication efficiency of PVM 15 was significantly higher than that of PVM J3666 (G_{J3666}65A) ($p <0.01$) but comparable to that of PVM J3666 (G_{J3666}65AU) ($p >0.05$) indicating that the level of G glycoprotein and/or some other viral factors played a significant role in the replication of the viruses in macrophage-like cells (Figure 19B).

Since PVM is a mouse pathogen and the RAW 264.7 cells were derived from mouse, there was the possibility that either inherent host factors or intrinsic properties of the macrophage-like cells mediated the observed attenuation. Therefore, to address these possibilities, the replication kinetics of the biological isolates were assayed in primary mouse embryonic fibroblast (MEF): wild type (C57BL/6) and interferon-alpha receptor deficient (C57BL/6.IFNAR$^{-/-}$). The MEF from C57BL/6.IFNAR$^{-/-}$ were included because the G protein of the related human metapneumovirus (hMPV) was reported to inhibit type-I interferon responses (Bao et al., 2008; Bao et al., 2013). Therefore, the effect of host intrinsic factors including the type-I interferon response on the replication pattern of the viruses could be studied.

In MEFs from C57BL/6, PVM J3666 (G_{J3666}65AU), PVM 15 and PVM J3666 (G_{J3666}65A) had a mean titre of 9.20 x 10^1 PFU/ml, 1.33 x 10^2 PFU/ml and 1.70 x 10^2 PFU/ml, respectively, on day 2 postinfection (Figure 20A). However, by day 4 postinfection, PVM J3666 (G_{J3666}65A) with a mean titre of 1.95 x 10^4 PFU/ml had replicated 2.6-fold higher than PVM 15 with a mean titre of 7.38 x 10^3 PFU/ml and PVM J3666 (G_{J3666}65AU) with an average titre of 7.4 x 10^3 PFU/ml. On day 7 postinfection, the differences in replication efficiency between PVM J3666 (G_{J3666}65A) at 7.45 x 10^5 PFU/ml and PVM J3666 (G_{J3666}65AU) at 2.14 x 10^5 PFU/ml or PVM 15 at 2.33 x 10^5 PFU/ml had increased to approximately 3.5-

fold. Statistical analysis showed that the mean titres of PVM J3666 (G_{J3666}65A) on day 4 ($p < 0.01$) and day 7 ($p < 0.05$) were significantly higher to that of PVM 15.

In MEFs from C57BL/6.IFNAR$^{-/-}$ mice, PVM 15, PVM J3666 (G_{J3666}65AU) and PVM J3666 (G_{J3666}65A) demonstrated equal replication efficiencies at days 1 and 2 postinfection. However, by day 4 postinfection, the mean titre of PVM J3666 (G_{J3666}65A) at 4.08 x 10^4 PFU/ml was 4-fold higher than the mean titres of PVM J3666 (G_{J3666}65AU) at 1.13 x 10^4 PFU/ml and PVM 15 at 1.02 x 10^4 PFU/ml. The 4-fold difference in replication kinetics was maintained until day 7 to produce a significant statistical difference between PVM J3666 (G_{J3666}65A) at 9.35 x 10^5 PFU/ml and PVM 15 at 2.26 x 10^5 PFU/ml.

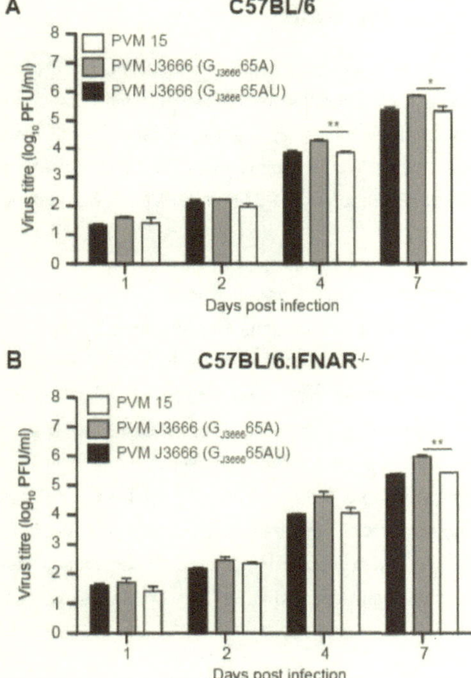

Figure 20: The attenuation of PVM J3666 (G_{J3666}65A) in RAW 264.7 cells is not host-specific and independent of type-I interferon.
Multi-cycle replication kinetics of PVM 15, PVM J3666 (G_{J3666}65A) and PVM J3666 (G_{J3666}65AU) in C57BL/6 MEF (A) or C57BL/6.IFNAR$^{-/-}$ MEF (B). Cells were infected at an MOI of 0.01 PFU/cell. At the indicated time points, cells and supernatants were collected and quantified by plaque assay on Vero cells under methylcellulose. Each data point represents the average value of two independent experiments performed in duplicates. The standard deviation between the runs is represented by the error bars. At each time point, one-way ANOVA followed by Dunnett's multiple comparison test were used to compare PVM J3666 (G_{J3666}65A) and PVM J3666 (G_{J3666}65AU) to PVM 15. Differences were considered significant at $p < 0.05$. (** $p \leq 0.01$).

In conclusion, the host specific factors and type-I interferon do not appear to affect the replication kinetics of the viruses in MEF suggesting that the G glycoprotein of PVM do not perform the same function as those of hMPV. This will imply that a yet to be identified intrinsic property of the RAW 264.7 cells restricted the replication of PVM J3666 (G_{J3666}65A) in the cells.

3.4 Recombinant PVMs encoding a N-terminus truncated G protein or lacking the G gene are attenuated in macrophage-like cells due to the level of their G glycoprotein expression

Concluding from the results of previous sections, the differing amount of G protein produced by infected cells was the most probable explanation for the functional differences among the viruses, whether recombinant or biological strains. Therefore, the experiments in this section were designed to retrospectively analyse if the findings would also extend to rPVM with truncated G (rPVM-Gt) or a mutant lacking the G gene (rPVM-ΔG-GFP). rPVM-ΔG-GFP and rPVM-Gt were attenuated in mice (Krempl et al., 2007)

rPVM-Gt was rescued from PVM 15/ ATCC background, the G gene was truncated by mutagenesis PCR that deleted 167 nucleotides that followed the 10 nucleotides of the gene start sequence thereby removing all the 5' UTR and first 32 coding codons in the normal G ORF. This mutation created a new 5' UTR of only 14 nucleotides and moved the second AUG from its initial position at codon 34 to become the first AUG in the G ORF (Krempl et al., 2007). The G protein of rPVM-Gt is accepted to be functionally similar to that of the attenuated PVM 15/ Warwick, containing a frameshift mutation that truncated the cytoplasmic domain of the translated G protein. rPVM-GFP-Gt is a variant of rPVM-Gt containing GFP gene as an additional gene immediately upstream of the G gene. rPVM-ΔG-GFP is a mutant of rPVM containing GFP in place of the naturally occurring G gene. These viruses were designed to allow the direct analysis of the role of the cytoplasmic portion of the G protein as well as the complete G protein on the properties of the virus (Krempl et al., 2007).

3.4.1 The level of G protein expression correlated with incorporation into virus particles

To analyse the effect of the truncation of the G gene in rPVM-Gt on G protein levels, the amount of G glycoprotein produced in BHK-21 cells infected with rPVM-Gt relative to rPVM at an MOI of 0.1 PFU/cell after 4 days was determined by Western blotting as previously described in section 3.2.2. The quantity of detectable G protein in rPVM-Gt-infected cells was significantly lower compared to rPVM-infected cells (Figure 21A). Normalization of the signal intensity of the G protein to the signal intensity of P protein showed that the quantity of G protein in rPVM-Gt-infected cells was 3-fold lower in comparison to cells infected with rPVM (Figure 21B).

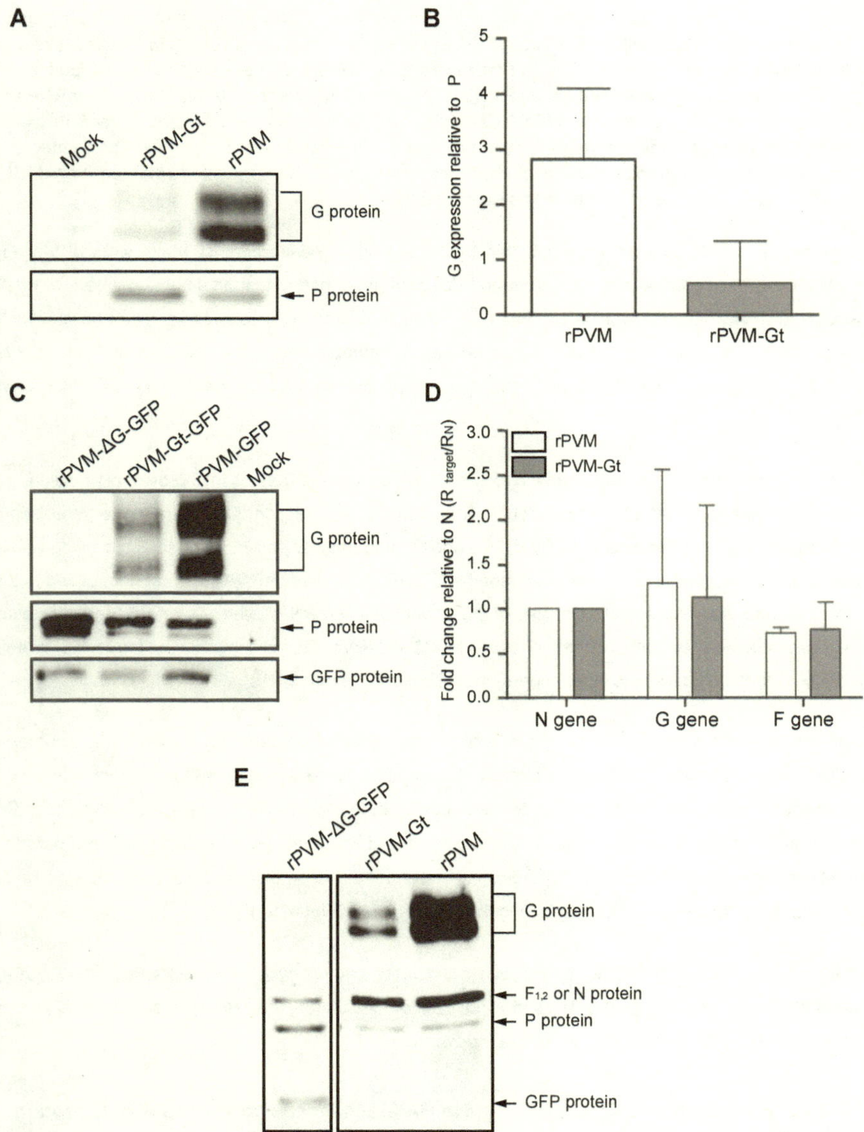

Figure 21: The rate of G protein expression by rPVM-Gt is reduced and correlated with the rate of G incorporation into virus particles.

(A) BHK-21 cells, mock infected or infected with rPVM or rPVM-Gt, were lysed at day 4 postinfection and subjected to Western blot analysis. PVM proteins were detected with antiserum from rPVM-infected convalescent mice combined with chemiluminescence imaging. (B). The signals of the G protein per lane were normalized to the corresponding signal of the P protein. Error bars represent the standard error between the four independent experiments. (C) Cells lysates were prepared from BHK-21 cells infected with the indicated GFP-expressing rPVM that were treated as described for

A. A representative of at four experiments is shown (D) Viral mRNA quantification by SYBR-green based qRT-PCR. Total cellular RNA from BHK-21 cells infected with rPVM or rPVM-Gt were reverse transcribed with random hexamers and subjected to qPCR with primers specific for the indicated mRNA. The data were analysed the LinRegPCR program (Ruijter et al., 2009). The target mRNA in each group was normalized to 18s rRNA as control then expressed as a fold change over N mRNA. Error bars represent the standard deviation between two independent experiments performed in triplicates. (E) Western blot analysis of virus protein incorporation into purified virus particles (MOI = 2 PFU/cell). The blot was prepared as described for A.

Since only P and G proteins were detected by the antiserum raised against whole virus, rPVM and rPVM-Gt expressing enhanced GFP from an additional gene inserted immediately upstream of the G gene, and rPVM-ΔG-GFP were also tested as above to use the GFP expression level as additional internal standard. The amount of GFP produced was comparable among the tested groups but the level of G protein was not, thus confirming reduced G protein expression in rPVM-Gt-infected cells (Figure 21C).

To exclude any alteration in gene transcription on the observed differences in G protein expression, the G-mRNA levels were determined by qRT-PCR as described in section 3.2.3. Due to the sequentially mechanism of gene transcription in PVM, two additional genes, N and F, were selected alongside to deduce events upstream and downstream of the G gene. Each viral mRNA was first normalized to the 18s rRNA and later expressed as a ratio of the normalized N mRNA levels. The mRNA quantification showed similar gene transcription rate between rPVM and rPVM-Gt, implying that the reduced G protein in rPVM-Gt infected-cells was independent of transcription (Figure 21D).

Lastly, the amount of G protein incorporated into virus particles was determined by subjecting a sucrose-purified virus preparation to Western blotting. The proteins were detected with antiserum from rPVM convalescent mice. The reduced G protein expression in rPVM-Gt-infected cells led to diminished G glycoprotein incorporation into virus particles collected at 48 hours postinfection when compared to rPVM particles prepared the same way indicating that G protein incorporation into virus particle is directly proportional to the amount of G available in the infected cells (Figure 21E).

These results highlighted above tallied with observations made with rPVM encoding the J3666-G variants and with the biological isolates of PVM 15 and PVM J3666, indicating the amount of G protein expressed on the PVM-infected cells is strain dependent.

3.4.2 The replication efficiency of PVM in RAW 264.7 cells correlated with G protein levels

The replication kinetic of biological isolates and rPVM mutants suggested a potential role for G protein in the replication efficiencies of the viruses in cell culture, especially in the macrophage-like cells. Therefore, to understand how G protein levels affect replication efficiencies *in vitro*, the following pairs of viruses: rPVM-Gt and rPVM; and rPVM-ΔG-GFP and rPVM-GFP were compared at MOI of 0.01 in BHK-21 cells, RAW 264.7 cells and MEFs from C57BL/6 and C57BL/6.IFNAR$^{-/-}$ mice. Confluent BHK-21 cells or MEF in 12-well plates or RAW 264.7 cells in 75 ml flask were infected in duplicates. At 24-

hour intervals post infection, supernatant aliquots were taken from RAW 264.7 cells and replaced with an equivalent volume of fresh medium while both cell-bound and cell-free viruses were collected from MEFs and BHK-21 cells.

The absence of G protein in rPVM-ΔG-GFP or 3-fold (75%) reduction in rPVM-Gt did not affect replication of the viruses in BHK-21 cells as the virus pairs replicated equally from the start to the end of the experiment (Figure 22A). rPVM-Gt replicated efficiently as rPVM to reach mean titres of approximately 1 x 10^7 PFU/ml at day 7 while rPVM-ΔG-GFP also replicated very similarly to rPVM-GFP to reach mean titres of 2.6 x 10^5 PFU/ml and 4 x 10^5 PFU/ml, respectively. This result revealed that replication of PVM in BHK-21 cells is indeed independent of the G gene as previously reported (Krempl et al., 2007).

On the other hand, there appeared to be a correlation between the level of G protein expression and replication efficiencies in RAW 264.7 cells with the caveat that G protein levels were quantified in BHK-21 cells. The replication efficiency decreased in the order of rPVM, rPVM-GFP, rPVM-Gt and rPVM-ΔG-GFP (Figure 22B). Obvious differences in growth kinetics were first noticed on day 2 with the GFP-expressing viruses when the mean titre of rPVM-ΔG-GFP at 1.16 x 10^2 PFU/ml was 50-fold lower than the mean titre of rPVM-GFP at 5.8 x 10^3 PFU/ml. The difference in growth efficiency between rPVM-ΔG-GFP (5.2 x 10^2 PFU/ml) and rPVM-GFP (7.3 x 10^4 PFU/ml) increased to about 140-fold on day 3 and then dropped on day 4 to about 70-fold (4.8 x 10^3 PFU/ml as against 3.4 x 10^5 PFU/ml). From this time-point on the difference in titres between rPVM-GFP and rPVM-ΔG-GFP increased gradually from 207-fold on day 5 to 415-fold on day 6 and finally to 500-fold on day 7. This difference was statistically significant ($p < 0.05$).

Noticeable difference in replication efficiency between rPVM-Gt and rPVM was first recorded at day 3 postinfection when the mean titre of rPVM-Gt at 6.9 x 10^3 PFU/ml was 18-fold lower than that of rPVM at 1.3 x 10^5 PFU/ml. The 18-fold replication difference was maintained until day 5: rPVM-Gt (1.2 x 10^5 PFU/ml) and rPVM (2 x 10^6 PFU/ml). By day 6, the difference in the mean titres dropped somewhat to 10 fold (5.6 x 10^5 PFU/ml for rPVM-Gt and 6 x 10^6 PFU/ml for rPVM) but increased again by day 7 to produce the maximum difference of 20-fold (rPVM-Gt at 5.3 x 10^5 PFU/ml against rPVM at 1 x 10^7 PFU/ml). Statistical analysis confirmed that the difference was not a chance occurrence ($p = 0.0004$). The differing extent of attenuation indicated that replication of PVM in RAW 264.7 cells is dependent of the amount of G protein produced by infected cells.

Next, due to the higher attenuation of rPVM-ΔG-GFP in RAW 264.7 cells compared to PVM J3666 (G_{J3666}65A), the replication kinetics was examined in MEF from C57BL/6 to exclude mouse intrinsic factors and MEF from C57BL/6.IFNAR$^{-/-}$ mice to eliminate the effect of interferon (IFN)- type I in the absence of the G protein as reported for the related hMPV (Bao et al., 2008; Bao et al., 2013). In MEF from C57BL/6, rPVM-ΔG-GFP replicated 10-fold more efficiently at all tested time points to reach a mean titre of 3.6 x 10^5 PFU/ml at day 7 compared to 4.3 x 10^4 PFU/ml recorded for rPVM-GFP (Figure 22C). A similar observation was made for MEF from C57BL/6.IFNAR$^{-/-}$, where rPVM-ΔG-GFP reached a mean titre of 6.2 x 10^5 PFU/ml on day 7 compared to 7.2 x 10^4 PFU/ml documented for rPVM-GFP

(Figure 22D). However, the differences in titres were only statistically significant on days 4 and 7 in MEF from C57BL/6.IFNAR$^{-/-}$ compared to MEF from C57BL/6 where the differences at all tested time points were statistically significant.

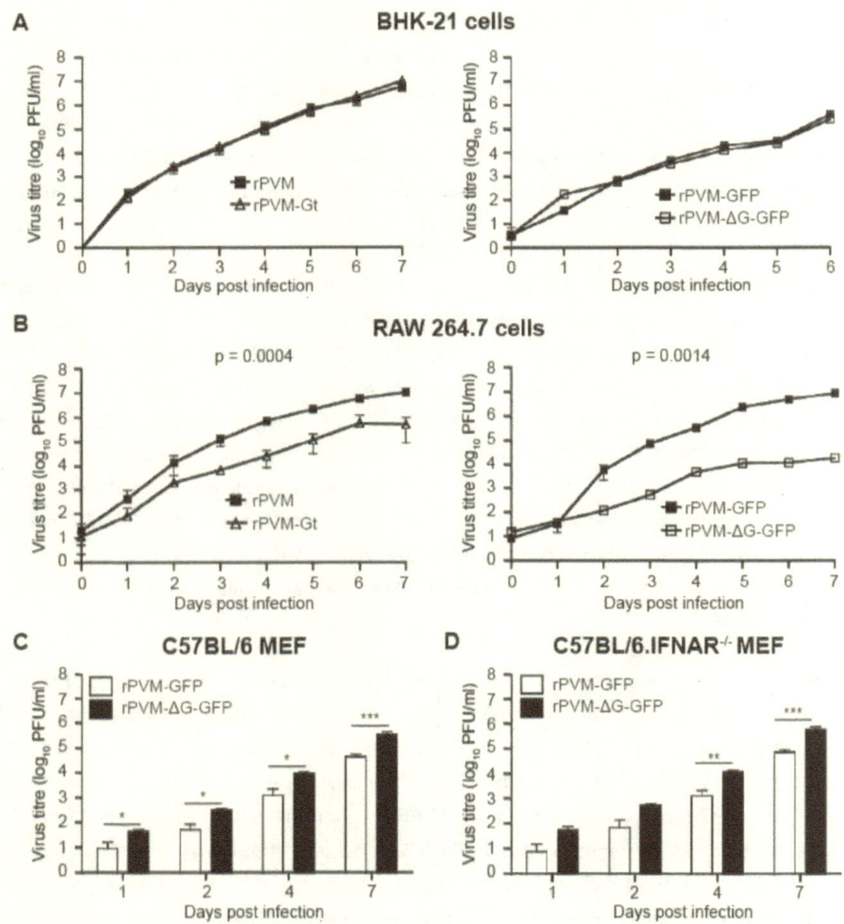

Figure 22: The rate of replication in RAW 264.7 cells appears to be proportional to the level of G glycoprotein expression.

Multi-cycle replication kinetics: (A) BHK-21 cells, (B) RAW 264.7 cells, and (C and D) MEFs were infected with either rPVM and rPVM-Gt or rPVM-GFP and rPVM-ΔG-GFP at MOI of 0.01 PFU/cell. At the indicated time points, cells and supernatants were harvested for BHK-21 cells and MEFs while supernatants were collected from RAW 264.7 cells. Virus titres were quantified by plaque assay on Vero cells. Data points represent mean values of two independent experiments performed in duplicates. Error bars indicate the standard deviation between the runs. A paired T test was used to test statistical significance between rPVM and rPVM-Gt pair and rPVM-GFP and rPVM-ΔG-GFP pair in the RAW 264.7 cells. The data from MEFs kinetics were analysed using the unpaired T test with Welch's correction. Differences were considered significant at $p < 0.05$ (** $p \leq 0.01$ and $p \leq 0.001$).

Lastly, a single-cycle replication assay was performed at MOI of 2 PFU/cell using rPVM-GFP, rPVM-GFP-Gt and rPVM-ΔG-GFP to determine whether higher infectious doses could abolish the negative effect of the G protein on replication kinetics in RAW 264.7 cells. During single-cycle replication, majority of the cells are thought to be infected at the beginning of the experiment leading to synchronous virus yield (Becker et al., 1992; Holder et al., 2011). Surprisingly, the viruses had comparable kinetics at all selected time points (Figure 23), signifying that the restriction of rPVM-GFP-Gt and rPVM-ΔG-GFP during multicycle replication was not a result of impaired entry into the cells but rather due to a restriction in virus spread in the absence of adequate amount of G protein.

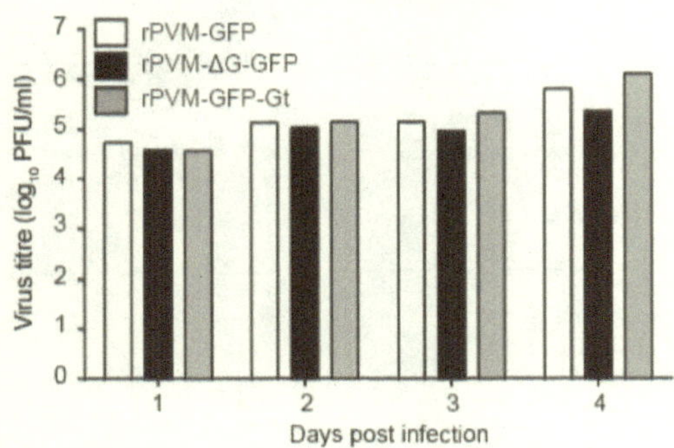

Figure 23: Attenuation of rPVM-ΔG-GFP and rPVM-GFP-Gt in RAW 264.7 is due to limited spread during multi-cycle replication.
Replication kinetics of GFP expressing viruses. Duplicate cultures of RAW 264.7 cells were infected with rPVM-GFP or rPVM-GFP-Gt or rPVM-ΔG-GFP at MOI of 2 PFU/cell. Supernatant aliquots were taken at the indicated time points and replaced with an equivalent volume of fresh medium. Viral titres were determined by plaque assay on Vero cells. The day 3 postinfection time point was prepared from a different independent experiments performed to confirm the results from days 1, 2 and 4 performed concomitantly.

3.4.3 Attenuation of rPVM-ΔG-GFP and rPVM-Gt is specific for macrophages

To determine whether the restriction of rPVM-Gt and rPVM-ΔG-GFP during the multicycle growth in RAW 264.7 cells was macrophage-specific, the growth kinetics of rPVM-GFP-Gt and rPVM-ΔG-GFP were compared against rPVM-GFP in bone marrow-derived macrophages from C57BL/6 mouse (C57BL/6 macrophages) at an MOI of 0.01 PFU/cell. Figure 24 shows the percentage of macrophage in collected bone marrow cells before and after differentiation with macrophage-colony stimulating factor (M-CSF). The marrows of the hind bones were collected into 50 ml polypropylene tubes containing RPMI-1640 medium supplemented with macrophage-colony stimulating factor (M-CSF) under sterile conditions. Thereafter, 3 x 10^6 cells were seeded per 100 mm Petri dish and incubated for 7 days at 32°C and 5% CO_2 with medium replacement on the second and fourth day. After 7 days, the differentiated cells were collected with 10% EDTA and stained with anti-CD11b, anti-F4/80 and live/dead fixable violet viability stain (Weischenfeldt and Porse, 2008).

A. Before differentiation with M-CSF

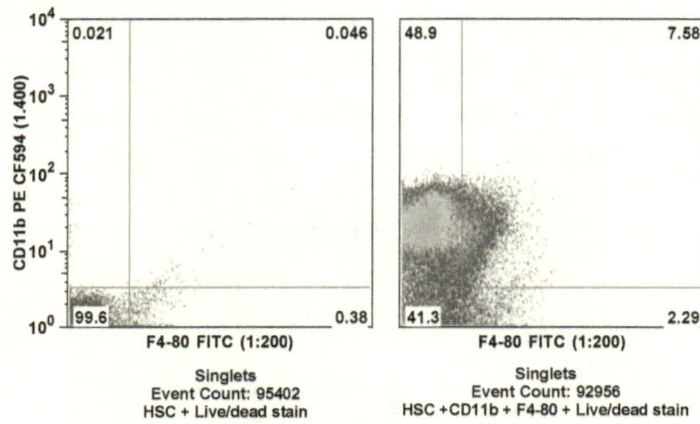

B. After differentiation with M-CSF

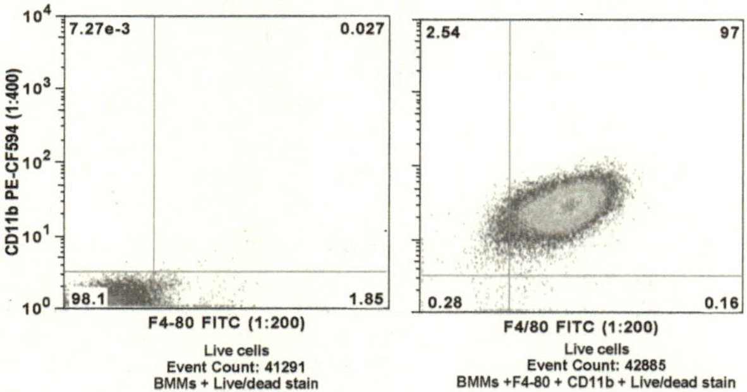

Figure 24: FACS staining of undifferentiated and differentiated BMMs.
Phenotypic characterization of undifferentiated BMMs (a) and differentiated BMMs (b) with live /dead fixable violet dead kit, F4/80 and CD11b. The undifferentiated BMMs were bone marrow cells stained directly after isolation while the differentiated BMMs were collected after 7 days treatment with M-CSF. The live cells were first gated as viable stain negative then the BMMs as F4/80 and CD11b double positive.

At day 1 postinfection, the growth of rPVM-GFP at 7 PFU/ml was equivalent to those of rPVM-GFP-Gt and rPVM-ΔG-GFP but by day 3 postinfection, the mean titre of rPVM-GFP rose to 1.5 x 10^3 PFU/ml while the mean titres of the other two viruses remained at 7 PFU/ml. On day 5, the mean titre of rPVM-GFP had increased by over 2000-fold from day 1 to reach a mean titre of 1.6 x 10^4 PFU/ml as against rPVM-GFP-Gt (mean titre of 57 PFU/ml) and rPVM-ΔG-GFP (mean titre of 30 PFU/ml) that increased marginally by 8-fold and 2.5-fold, respectively. On day 7, the average titre of rPVM-GFP was 4.9 x 10^4 PFU/ml in comparison to 70 PFU/ml recorded for rPVM-GFP-Gt and 43 PFU/ml noted for rPVM-ΔG-GFP, to produce a fold difference of 700 and 1100, respectively, (Figure 25). Thus, it was confirmed that the restriction of rPVM-Gt and rPVM-ΔG-GFP during the multicycle growth in RAW 264.7 cells was not specific for RAW 264.7 cells but for macrophage-like cells. Furthermore, the restriction was more pronounced in primary macrophages than in RAW 264.7 cell.

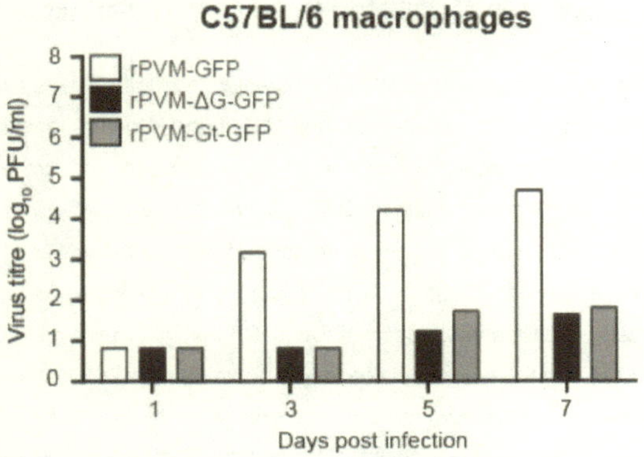

Figure 25: Attenuation in RAW 264.7 cells is macrophage-specific.
Replication kinetics of GFP-expressing viruses. Duplicate cultures of C57BL/6 macrophages in 6-well plates were infected with rPVM-GFP, rPVM-GFP-Gt and rPVM-ΔG-GFP at MOI of 0.01 PFU/cell. Cells and supernatants were harvested at indicated time points, clarified by centrifugation and titrated by plaque assay on Vero cells. The mean titres ($\log_{10}$ PFU/ml) for one representative of two independent experiments are shown.

4. Discussion

4.1 The quasispecies of PVM J3666 represents two distinct populations

The clonal analysis of the quasispecies of PVM J3666 revealed that it represents a mixture of two distinct populations distinguishable by the composition of their G, SH and M genes: one population encodes a G gene, herein referred to as G_{J3666}65A, in which a short upstream open reading frame (uORF) precedes the main G ORF, and an SH gene containing an ORF that would be translated into a polypeptide of 114 amino acids. In the second population, the SH gene codes for a polypeptide of 92 amino acids. In the case of the G gene here termed G_{J3666}65U, a point mutation involving the exchange of adenine at nucleotide 65 to uridine ablates the stop codon of the uORF fusing it to the main ORF, resulting in the extension of the main ORF and the corresponding length of the putative cytoplasmic tail of the translated G protein by 18 amino acids. The seven nucleotides differences between the M genes of G_{J3666}65A and G_{J3666}65U populations were within the untranslated region and affected the composition of the gene end signal.

Variability of the SH and G genes of PVM strain J3666 has been previously reported and was suggested to represent the quasispecies nature of the virus (Krempl and Collins, 2004; Thorpe and Easton, 2005). Here, analysis of 45 distinct clones showed that the virus preparation contained both forms of G gene (G_{J3666}65A and G_{J3666}65U) with a percentage distribution of almost 1:1. In addition, homogenous polymorphisms consisting entirely of either adenine or guanine at 7 nucleotides within the last 30 bases of the M gene and at 27 positions spread across the entire SH gene were identified. The polymorphisms in the M and SH genes clustered with the three distinct polymorphic bases that defined the G genes and together can be assigned to either the G_{J3666}65U or G_{J3666}65A clones. This present study revealed that the observed overlapping peaks within the assembled consensus sequence of RT-PCR products analysed in previous studies (Krempl and Collins, 2004; Thorpe and Easton, 2005) actually represent two distinct virus populations coexisting together and are not a reflection of the quasispecies nature of PVM strain J3666 as formerly suggested.

Whilst the percentage distribution of the populations in the virus preparation analysed might be explicit for this study, the heterogeneity of strain J3666 is not likely to be specific for the virus preparation used. Although, PVM J3666 was reported to originate from the same laboratory as reference strain 15 (Cook et al., 1998). The isolation history of PVM J3666 remains ambiguous. PVM J3666 was first described in 1995, almost 60 years after its likely isolation, when the sequence composition of its G gene was compared to that of an attenuated variant of PVM 15 (Randhawa et al., 1995). Consequently, all stocks of strain J3666 currently available in the different laboratories are traceable to this same source. In particular, eight of the 27 polymorphic positions of the SH gene identified in this work, that is, nucleotides 44, 70, 269, 283, 287, 292, 293 and 299 were also reported to be variable by previous independent study (Thorpe and Easton, 2005). This also included the size plasticity of the SH protein for 92 or 114 amino acids (Thorpe and Easton, 2005), as well as a variability of nucleotide positions, 65,104, 165 and

1121 of the G gene (Krempl and Collins, 2004). All the studies mentioned (Randhawa et al., 1995; Krempl and Collins, 2004; Thorpe and Easton, 2005) focused on determining the consensus sequence by direct analysis of RT-PCR products from RNA, which might explain why the additional polymorphisms detected in this present work might have been overlooked, especially since it was impossible to segregate the polymorphisms without cloning the RT-PCR products.

The composition of PVM J366 stocks may differ significantly between laboratories depending on the passage history and procedure. In support of this view, sequential passage of the mixed PVM J3666 preparation in BHK-21 cells eventually selected for the G_{J3666}65A population in one of two independent experiments, further indicating an effect of handling technique on the percentage composition of the virus. In addition, it is noteworthy that the original sequence analysis assigning the nucleotide 65A structure to the J3666-G gene involved amplification of the virus in BS-C-1 cells (Randhawa et al., 1995), whereas the study that first identified the G_{J3666}65U-G gene suggesting it as the major J3666-G gene variant was based on RT-PCR products derived from post-mortem mouse lungs samples (Krempl and Collins, 2004).

There are two possible explanations to the origin of the G_{J3666}65A and G_{J3666}65U populations within PVM J3666. The first probable explanation is that PVM J3666 originating from the laboratory that first described PVM, was accidentally contaminated with another isolate during its isolation history. For instance, eleven distinct isolates were originally isolated and characterized concomitantly by the researchers that first described PVM (Horsfall and Hahn, 1939; Horsfall and Hahn, 1940). Also, none of these studies explicitly mentioned J3666, which when coupled with the limited information on the isolation history and the lost years between the time of its supposed isolation and re-emergence makes it difficult to trace the origin retrospectively. The second possible explanation is that one of the populations evolved from the other during passaging of the original J3666 strain in either BS-C-1 cells or mice. Horsfall and Hahn (Horsfall and Hahn, 1940) reported that the isolate 15 now referred to as PVM 15 was not initially virulent for mice, but acquired virulence as it was serially passaged in mouse lungs. Interestingly, the PVM 15-SH ORF encodes a polypeptide of 92 amino acids, with almost similar amino acids composition, as found in the PVM G_{J3666}65U population. In addition, the length of SH ORF (92 amino acids) and G ORF (414 amino acids) of the PVM G_{J3666}65U population are similar to those of PVM Y, a strain isolated from a natural outbreak in nude mice (Weir et. al., 1988; NLM Acc.No. JQ899033.1) and of canine pneumovirus, CnPnV, isolated from diseased dog (Renshaw et al., 2010). These similarities suggest that the G_{J3666}65A might be the parent population and the G_{J3666}65U population evolved as the virus was being passaged in mouse lungs (Cook et al., 1998) as previously described for PVM 15 (Horsfall and Hahn, 1940).

BS-C-1 cells are derived from kidney cells of the African green monkey (Hopps et al., 1963) and have been reported to be somewhat restrictive for PVM replication (Miyata et al., 1995; Dyer et al., 2007). The plaque purification and subsequent propagation of PVM 15 in BS-C-1 cells had been suggested to select for an attenuated variant referred to as PVM 15/Warwick (Krempl and Collins, 2004). Consequently, there is a possibility that the limited propagation of PVM J3666 in BS-C-1 cells led to the selection and subsequent amplification of a new population over time. Furthermore, the finding that the nucleotide differences between the SH and M genes of the G_{J3666}65A population and G_{J3666}65U population involved A → G transition pointing to a biased hypermutation event, which will suggest the selection of the less pathogenic variant (G_{J3666}65A population) from the more virulent variant (G_{J3666}65U population). Of note, the serial passaging of an isolate (Ane4) of CnPnV in canine fibroblast A72 cells led to selection of a new population termed Brne17 (Renshaw et al., 2010). In addition to other mutations, Renshaw and colleagues showed that the G protein of the Brne17 was truncated at carboxyl terminus due to a point mutation that was selected at the third passage but became dominant at passage 17 (Renshaw et al., 2011). Also, the passaging of PVM 15 in BHK-21 cells and chick-embryo Tyrode tissue-culture medium, was associated with reduced virulence in mice indicative of a selection event (Horsfall and Hahn, 1940; Shimonaski and Came, 1970). In line with this, the G_{J3666}65A population was tentatively assumed to be the variant selected during the passaging of the original PVM J3666 stock in cell culture, since it was also possible in this study to select a population exclusively containing a G gene with nucleotide 65A structure during the serial passaging of the mixed stock, although this involved BHK-21 cells rather than BS-C-1 cells. Interestingly, this form of biased hypermutation observed between the SH and M genes of G_{J3666}65U and G_{J3666}65A populations resembled an A → G transition identified in the matrix gene of pathogenic strains of measles virus that became defective during the establishment of persistent infection in the brain (Cattaneo et al., 1988; Cattaneo et al., 1989; Wong et al., 1991) and selection of RSV anti-G escape mutants (Rueda et al., 1994; Walsh et al., 1998). However, unlike with the measles virus, the A → G hypermutation in the anti-RSV G escape mutants did not affect the replication efficiencies of the mutants in HEp-2 cells (Rueda et al., 1994; Walsh et al., 1998).

4.2 Influence of the 5' untranslated region on G protein expression

The present study revealed that expression levels of G protein vary depending on the PVM strain, respective isolate or on the specific G gene organization. This modulation occurred on translational level mediated by the structure and organization of the 5' untranslated region (UTR) of the PVM G gene

The generation of the rPVM-G_{J3666}65A and rPVM-G_{J3666}65U differing exclusively by the G genes permitted the association of differences in the level of G protein expression to the presence of the uORF within the 5' UTR of G_{J3666}65A and the extension of the main ORF in G_{J3666}65U. G protein levels expressed by rPVM-G_{J3666}65A-infected cells were approximately 40% reduced relative to the G protein levels expressed in strain-15 infected cells. In contrast, the extension of the G_{J3666}65U main ORF by 54 nucleotides coding for additional 18 amino acids due to the merging of the uORF to the downstream ORF increased the level of G glycoprotein expressed in infected BHK-21 cells by 50% relative to strain 15-infected cells. Extending these observations to the biological strains (PVM 15 vs PVM J3666 (G_{J3666}65A)) showed that G expression was almost 50% reduced in PVM J3666 (G_{J3666}65A)-infected cells as observed with rPVM-G_{J3666}65A. On the other hand, the G protein level was only 17% reduced in cells infected with the mixed PVM J3666 (G_{J3666}65AU) expressing both G_{J3666}65A and G_{J3666}65U at almost a ratio of 1:1. This indicates that the increased G expression by G_{J3666}65U compensated for the negative effect of G_{J3666}65A. Subsequent analysis of PVM-specific transcripts (N, G and F mRNAs) from

BHK-21 cells infected with the different viruses provided the direct evidence for modulation at translational level or post-transcription stage since variation in the level of G protein expression was neither accompanied by disparity in G mRNA level nor in that of the upstream (N mRNA) or downstream (F mRNA) gene.

Of note, nucleotide 30G (genomic sense) in the 5' UTR of the G-strain 15 gene ablates the start codon of the uORF. Thus, the absence of this uORF represents the major structural difference between rPVM and rPVM-G_{J3666}65A. There are additional four amino acids differences between the G-strain 15 and G_{J3666}65A, that is, L5F, V28G, T112A and T347S, but it is unlikely that these substitutions contributed to the reduced G expression noted for G_{J3666}65A. Moreover, quantification of G protein levels in mutants of rPVM-G_{J3666}65A containing threonine at amino acids 112 and 347 showed both substitutions either singly or together do not affect G protein expression (A. Adenugba A. and C. Krempl, unpublished observations). Therefore, the presence of uORF before the main ORF of G_{J3666}65A was suggested to be responsible for the reduced expression of detectable G protein in rPVM-G_{J3666}65A-infected cells compared to cells infected with rPVM. The presence of uORFs and other secondary structures within the 5' UTR have been shown to modulate the level of protein synthesis from the main ORF by diverting ribosomes from the downstream main ORF (reviewed in Barbosa et al., 2013). The G genes of all strains of human RSV sequenced so far contain an upstream ORF starting eight nucleotides upstream of the G ORF within the gene-start signal sequence. This uORF overlaps the main G ORF and encodes a polypeptide of 15 amino acids (Wertz et al., 1985). Teng et. al., (Teng et al., 2001) showed that the ablation of AUG of this uORF increased the translation efficiency of the main RSV G ORF. In another artificial system involving the transfection of a dicistronic mRNA construct into plant protoplast, the translation of the first primary ORF located 18 nucleotides downstream of the uORF as found in G_{J3666}65A was inhibited by the uORF preceding it (Futterer and Hohn, 1992).

In the case of G_{J3666}65U, ablation of the stop codon connects the uORF to the downstream ORF creating a new G ORF potentially initiating translation from AUG_{29} instead of AUG_{83}. This arrangement would extend the putative cytoplasmic tail of G by 18 amino acids and, at the same time, correlated with increased levels of G protein in cells infected with rPVM-G_{J3666}65U compared to the other two rPVMs. The close proximity of AUG_{29} to the cap region should not affect G protein translation since protein translation by scanning mechanism was not affected by the distance between the cap and the first AUG in yeast mRNA (Berthelot et al., 2004). However, the AUG_{29} is in a weak translational initiation context (CAA<u>AUG</u>A, AUG_{29} is underlined) suggesting that an appreciable quantity of ribosomes might slip by to initiate translation of the majority of G_{J3666}65U protein at the downstream AUG_{83} (AGU<u>AUG</u>G, AUG_{83} underlined) that is in a more optimal Kozak context. The resulting protein would rather match the G protein of strain 15. Thus, polypeptides initiated at AUG_{29} would add up to the majority of polypeptides initiated at the downstream AUG, consequently increasing the overall amount of G produced. This is of importance since the only PVM strain, PVM Y (Weir et al., 1988; NLM Acc. No. JQ899033), isolated from an natural outbreak in a housing facility and the related canine pneumovirus (CnPnV) isolated from diseased dogs (Decaro et al., 2014; Renshaw et al., 2010) contain a G gene encoding an extended main ORF comparable to G_{J3666}65U. Hence, extended G ORF and upregulated expression of G may be a hallmark of natural PVM strains and related species.

To complement the studies addressing the extension of the G ORF another construct, rPVM-Gt, was included that encoded a G protein lacking the cytoplasmic tail (Krempl et al., 2007). This virus had displayed an attenuated pathology phenotype in mice that appeared to be replication independent. Surprisingly, Western blot analysis of BHK-21 cells infected with rPVM-Gt revealed a 75% reduction in the quantity of G protein relative to G-strain 15 protein expressed from rPVM. In addition, when purified particles of rPVM-Gt and rPVM were analysed the incorporation of G glycoprotein into these virions correlated with the G protein amount expressed by the infected cells. Since the previous study (Krempl et al., 2007) just addressed the general expression, overall incorporation and eventual secretion of G but did not perform quantitative analysis, the results were unexpected. However, for the distantly related influenza virus, the deletion of the cytoplasmic tail of the neuraminidase protein was also associated with almost 50% reduction in neuraminidase expression by infected cells that subsequently resulted into its decrease incorporation into infectious virions (Garcia-Sastre and Palese, 1995; Mitnaul et al., 1996).

There are two possible mechanisms for the reduced expression and incorporation levels of Gt. First, the cytoplasmic tail of the PVM-G affected the correct processing, transport and stability, respective turnover of the protein and hence its efficient overall expression in infected cells. This would be in line with results of functional analyses of the role of cytoplasmic tail of several type-II glycoproteins found in enveloped RNA viruses either via direct expression from the genome of recombinant viruses or in artificial systems. These studies showed that the cytoplasmic domain of different type-II glycoproteins was required for adequate processing and/or intracellular transport of the glycoprotein to the cell surface (Spriggs and Collins, 1990; Wilson et al., 1990; Garcia-Sastre and Palese, 1995; Schmitt et al., 1999).

As for a second possible mechanism, the reduced expression levels of the G protein are determined by the translational initiation context of the shifted AUG of the major ORF. Similar to the structure of the RSV-G ORF, translation of the PVM strain 15 can potentially be initiated at two in-frame start codons, that is, AUG_{82} and AUG_{182}. Translational initiation at the downstream AUG_{182} would result in an N-terminally truncated G protein lacking the cytoplasmic portion. In order to force synthesis of G in direction to the truncated G, the Gt gene was generated by mutagenesis PCR that deleted 167 nucleotides after the 10 nucleotides gene start sequence thereby removing all of the 5' UTR and the first 32 codons of the regular G ORF (Krempl et al., 2007). This deletion created a new 5' UTR of only 14 nucleotides and moved the second AUG_{182} to the primary start codon, however, leaving its original rather unfavourable translational initiation context (CAA<u>AUG</u>U) untouched. Thus, reduced protein levels may be the result of a start codon in a suboptimal sequence place in rather short distance to the ribosomal binding site (reviewed by Kozak, 2005). Also, a combination of both mechanisms, i.e. dependence of correct synthesis and transport of G on the cytoplasmic portion, and inefficient translational initiation are conceivable. However, the determination of the exact mechanism would require further experimentation.

4.3 The effects of G expression levels on replication in cultured cells

In this work, the replication efficiency of PVM in macrophage-like cells, but not in other cell types, appeared to be dependent on the level of PVM-G protein expressed. A G-dependent replication restricting effect appears at least to involve assembly and release of virus particles from infected cells

The replication efficiency of rPVM-Gt, that was in parallel accompanied by a 75% reduction in G protein expression (Gt against G-strain 15), was 20-fold reduced relative to rPVM in macrophage-like RAW 264.7 cells while the complete absence of the G protein in rPVM-ΔG-GFP correlated with a 500-fold reduction in virus yield. This suggested that the quantity of G protein expressed was directly proportional to the replication efficiency in infected RAW 264.7 cells. This has to be taken with the caveat, that G expression was determined in BHK-21 cells, not RAW 264.7. The results are in line with a 50% decrease in G expression by PVM J3666 (G_{J3666}65A)-infected cells that correlated with an attenuated replication efficiency in RAW 264.7 cells. However, a 17% reduction in the quantity of G protein in biological PVM J3666 (G_{J3666}65AU)-infected cells appeared not to affect virus yield, neither did a 40% reduction in G expression the case of rPVM-G_{J3666}65A implying that a G protein reduction of more than 50 % observed in BHK-21-cell is required to observe an effect on replication efficiency in RAW 264.7 cells. On the other hand, an increase in available G protein levels in the case of rPVM-G_{J3666}65U appeared not to affect replication efficiency. This appears in line with the lack of effect of increasing RSV-G protein levels by deletion of the uORF on replication in HEp-2 cells that are otherwise sensitive to lack of G (Teng et al., 2001). Thus, a threshold amount of G appears to be required for efficient replication of PVM in RAW 264.7 cells, whereas overexpression has no influence.

Attenuation of replication in RAW 264.7 cells was only observed during multi-cycle replication experiments, at least for rPVM-Gt and rPVM-ΔG. Infected cells produced comparable virus yields as infection with wild-type rPVM during a single-cycle replication experiment (Figure 23; similar results were obtained using cell-free viruses or cell-associated viruses). In the experiment, GFP-expression in infected cells could be used as indicator for entry and transcription efficiency since rPVM-GFP based viruses were used. Since no differences in GFP-expression patterns were observed (data not shown) a limiting phase is likely to be at a late stage of the infectious cycle, for instance during morphogenesis or release from cell, events that would add up during the multi-cycle replication. Experiments directly addressing binding and entry into cells were not performed and an influence of G to this stage of infection cannot be excluded.

The attenuation of PVM mutants with debilitated or lacking G expression in macrophage-like cells is reminiscent of the phenotype of rRSV lacking the G gene. The absence of G in RSV has been implicated in a reduced replication efficiency in HEp-2 cells as opposed to Vero cells where G was completely dispensable (Techaarpornkul et al., 2001; Teng et al., 2001). Teng and co-workers (Teng et al., 2001) attributed the reduced replication efficiency to decreased infectivity coupled with some minor impairment during morphogenesis in the absence of G protein that was confirmed by Techaarpornkul and colleagues (Techaarpornkul et al., 2001) that studied the role of G protein in binding efficiency to glycosaminoglycans (GAG), a receptor for RSV during the infection phase (Krusat and Streckert, 1997;

Bourgeois et al., 1998; Hallak et al., 2000a; Hallak et al., 2000b). Although a receptor for PVM is not known, there appears to be significant functional similarities consequently implying comparable mechanisms. The results presented in this study are also in agreement with findings from analysis of replication kinetics of bRSV lacking the G gene in macrophages or peripheral blood lymphocytes that reported a fourfold increase in replication as well as spread of the virus in the presence of G protein (Schlender et al., 2003). Furthermore, alveolar macrophages were recently found to be one of the major sites of replication and production of infectious virions in rk2-PVM (expressing G_{J3666}65A protein variant) infected BALB/c mice (Dyer et al., 2015). Therefore, the increased infectivity of macrophages conferred by the G protein appears to be an additional virulence factor and might account for some of the difference in pathogenicity associated with the virulent and avirulent PVM strains.

Reduced growth efficiencies of rPVM-ΔG-GFP and rPVM-Gt in bone marrow-derived primary macrophages, but not in MEF or BHK-21 cells, suggested that the noted G level-dependent differences in replication were macrophage specific rather than species specific. The replication efficiencies of rPVM-Gt and rPVM-ΔG-GFP in BHK-21 cells were comparable to that of wild-type rPVM as previously reported (Krempl et al., 2007). This was regardless of the 75% reduction of G expression in rPVM-Gt-infected BHK-21 cells and of the complete absence of G protein in rPVM-ΔG-GFP-infected BHK-21 cells. Likewise, the 40% decrease in G expression in rPVM-G_{J3666}65A-infected or the 50 % decrease in PVM J3666 (G_{J3666}65A)-infected cells did not negatively affect the replication efficiency of the viruses. Rather the opposite was the case since the replication efficiency compared to the wild-type virus was increased (see below). Similar results were observed for PVM J3666 (G_{J3666}65A)- or rPVM-ΔG-infected MEF indicating that reduced G protein expression did not restrict replication in this two cell lines. It was unexpected that rPVM-G_{J3666}65A and PVM J3666 (G_{J3666}65A) replicated more efficiently than rPVM in BHK-21 cells, and PVM J3666 (G_{J3666}65A) than PVM 15 in MEFs. This increase in replication efficiency in BHK-21 cells is not easily assigned to the G protein since replication of rPVM lacking the G gene or of rPVM-Gt is unaffected in this cell line. The presence of uORF within 5'-UTR of G_{J3666}65A represents the major structural difference between rPVM and rPVM-G_{J3666}65A, hence the enhanced replication efficiency of rPVM-G_{J3666}65A in BHK-21 cells is possibly due to the uORF rather than the G protein levels. This improved replication conferred by the presence of the uORF may explain why PVM J3666 (G_{J3666}65A) population was selected from the mixed PVM J3666 stock during one of two sequential passaging experiments in BHK-21 cells. The growth efficiency of the selected PVM J3666 (G_{J3666}65A) was also higher than PVM 15 and the margin between the titres of the viruses at the end were greater than at the beginning. The deletion of the uORF in the L gene of Zaire ebolavirus was reported to negatively affect replication of the recombinant virus that was accompanied by reduced global viral RNA and mRNA synthesis (Shabman et al., 2013). The uORF was shown to directly contribute to L expression and hence the maintenance of viral replication during cellular stress (Shabman et al., 2013). This appears not to be the case here since the mRNA levels of the G_{J3666}65A is comparable to that of G-strain 15 mRNA as shown in Figure 14 and the role of G protein is not central to the virus replication and transcription as the L gene. Furthermore, the fact that the uORF appeared to contribute to growth kinetics at later point may suggest a direct contribution of a product translated from the uORF that accumulated during infection and contributed to the increase in virus titre as previously suggested for leader peptide produced from intraleader open reading frame of bovine coronavirus (Hofmann et al., 1993). Hofmann and colleagues (Hofmann et al., 1993) suggested that the downregulation of the virus proteins by the peptide from the uORF within the leader region of the mutant associated with persistence infection was responsible for its reduced replication compared to the wild-type parent lacking the uORF associated with acute infection. On the other hand, deletion of G correlated with enhanced replication in MEF implying a direct and rather negative role of G. Thus, there is presently no valid explanation for the enhanced replication efficiency conferred by lack of the uORF in some cells.

4.4 The effect of G expression level on virulence and replication in vivo

The G gene variants of the two PVM J3666 subpopulations; G_{J3666}65U and G_{J3666}65A, modulate the virulence of the rPVM mutants expressing them. Moreover, this difference in pathological properties appears majorly conferred by the expression levels of the G protein.

When the pathogenicity of rPVM-G_{J3666}65U and rPVM-G_{J3666}65A was analysed relative to rPVM, rPVM-G_{J3666}65U-infected mice lost more weight than rPVM-infected mice whereas the rPVM-G_{J3666}65A-infected mice hardly lost any weight. In addition, rPVM-G_{J3666}65A-infected mice were not diseased whereas rPVM-G_{J3666}65U-infected mice showed more symptoms such as ruffled fur, laboured breathing, and reduced activity than rPVM-infected mice (data not shown). The variations in virulence were attributed to the differences in the 5' UTR of the G genes of the viruses since these represent the single major differences between the recombinant viruses as discussed in 4.2 in detail. These differences in the 5'UTR were associated with the amount of protein expressed in BHK-21 cells as noted. Consequently, it is tempting to assume that it is the amount of G expressed that determines the pathogenicity, although, the quantities of G protein expressed by the infected lungs were not determined.

When the replication efficiencies of rPVM-G_{J3666}65U, rPVM-G_{J3666}65A and rPVM were evaluated in the lungs of BALB/c mice, all the three viruses had comparable titres at the peak of infection (day 6 postinfection) but the average titre in rPVM-G_{J3666}65U-infected mice was about 2-fold higher than the titre in mice infected with rPVM or rPVM-G_{J3666}65A at day 3 postinfection. This increased titre of rPVM-G_{J3666}65U over rPVM during the amplification phase may suggest an effect of the G protein on replication efficiency that contributed to the heightened virulence of rPVM-G_{J3666}65U. This effect is determinable only in the more sensitive natural infection system since increase in G levels did not influence replication in cultured cells (see 4.3). This is somewhat similar to previous RSV studies in which increased virus titres at early time points of the infection in BALB/c mice were associated with increased virulence (Moore et al., 2009; Stokes et al., 2013). In one instance, a higher viral load at day 1 postinfection in BALB/c mice infected with rRSV A2-2-20F, a recombinant RSV A2 strain expressing F protein gene from a clinical isolate A2001/2-20, correlated with more lung damage compared to RSV A2-infected mice (Stokes et al., 2013). In another study, increased kinetics and virus load by rRSV-A2-line 19F, a recombinant RSV A2 expressing line 19 F protein, during the amplification stage, that is, between days 0 and 4 postinfection was shown to cause more lung dysfunction compared to BALB/c mice infected with RSV A2 (Moore et al., 2009). In addition, for many RNA viruses such as influenza virus (Boon et al., 2011; Hatta et al., 2010; Liu et al., 2015) and lymphocytic choriomeningitis virus (Sullivan et al. 2015), higher replication at early time point was implicated as a mechanism of outpacing the innate immune response, thereby increasing the pathogenicity of the viruses over others with reduced replication kinetics. Nonetheless, further experiments are still required to determine the specific mechanism by which the increase G expression contributed to faster replication at the amplification stage.

The results regarding the differing virulence of rPVM and rPVM-G_{J3666}65U confirmed previous statements concerning an increased virulence of PVM J3666 compared to PVM 15 (Ellis et al., 2007; reviewed by Rosenberg and Domachowske, 2008), although data of a direct comparison was not provided. This was ascribed to a passage history of PVM J3666 in mice, whereas PVM strain 15 had been continuously been passaged in tissue culture. However, in the present study, this heightened virulence would rather be specific for the biological PVM J3666 population expressing the G_{J3666}65U variant than for the population expressing G_{J3666}65A that was originally assigned to PVM J3666. In the biological mixed PVM J3666 population, continuous passage in combination with a somewhat accelerated replication kinetics in mice may have favoured the G_{J3666}65U-containing population as discussed in 4.1 thus, explaining the observation of differing virulence between the strains.

The almost equal virus titres at the peak of virus replication on day 6 postinfection were somewhat reminiscent of the findings of Krempl and colleagues (Krempl et al., 2007) for rPVM-Gt and rPVM. An undistinguishable virus load of rPVM-Gt compared to rPVM on day 6, although earlier time points were not been investigated, correlated with an otherwise attenuated phenotype that consequently was suggested as being replication independent. The authors concluded that the cytoplasmic tail of the G protein affected pathogenesis independent of virus kinetics. Also, the study did not determine the amount of G expressed by rPVM-Gt nor noticed that rPVM-Gt expressed less amount of G than rPVM (see section 3.4.1). The results presented here for the rPVM-G_{J3666}65A and rPVM-G_{J3666}65U suggests that the attenuation of rPVM-Gt may correlate with expression levels of G rather than a direct effect of the absence of the cytoplasmic tail. Thus, the present study continued and extended previous data by providing an indication of a mechanism.

In summary, the in-vivo results supported the indication that the subpopulation with the G_{J3666}65U gene has a more favourable replication kinetics in mice. Furthermore, the analysis of the different PVM-G variants indicated that the amount of G protein expressed affected the degree of virulence in mice. This finding is different from previous studies (Karron et al., 1997; Teng et al., 2001; Schmidt et al., 2002; Krempl et al., 2007; Widjojoatmodjo et al., 2010) that addressed the effects of absence or presence of the G protein from BRSV, human RSV, and PVM in natural hosts or experimental animal models. In all these cases, the G-deletion mutants were highly attenuated indicating that the function of G within the pneumoviruses is conserved. This newly identified role of the G protein will require further experiments to identify how it contributes directly to pathogenicity.

5. Conclusion and perspective

The experiments described in this book showed the following:

1. The literature described PVM strain J3666 that is used in the research community is a mixture of two distinct populations, here termed PVM J3666 (G_{J3666}65A) and PVM J3666 (G_{J3666}65U), defined by distinct sequences and organizations of the M, SH and G genes. The possibility of selecting one of the population over the other during consecutive passaging was demonstrated by the isolation of the G_{J3666}65A population after seven consecutive passages in BHK-21 cells.
2. A major determinant of the PVM J3666 populations as well as of the reference strain PVM 15 is the organization of the 5' untranslated region (UTR) of the G genes. The presence of a small uORF within the 5' UTR of G_{J3666}65A and the extension of the ORF in G_{J3666}65U were associated with reduced and increased G protein expression, respectively, compared to an intermediate expression from the $G_{strain\ 15}$ gene that lacks an uORF. This difference in G protein expression occurred post-transcriptionally, as equal G-mRNA levels were detected in infected cells identifying a relatively new mechanism for negative stranded RNA viruses to regulate protein expression. In addition, the absence of the cytoplasmic tail in the G protein correlated with reduced G protein expression in infected-BHK-21 cells.
3. The level of G protein modulated the replication of PVM strains in macrophage-like cells. In addition, the organization of the 5'UTR and, thus, the expression level of the G protein influenced the overall virulence in mice as demonstrated by the generation of recombinant PVM containing the G_{J3666}65A or G_{J3666}65U genes.

To fully exclude influences of single amino acid polymorphisms between the G proteins of PVM strains, additional experiments are required, e.g. to check if deletion of the uORF in G_{J3666}65A gene will restore the amount of G protein expressed to comparable levels expressed from the G-strain 15 gene. Also, whether an extension of the main ORF of the G-strain 15 gene that is comparable to the structure of the G_{J3666}65U ORF will lead to an increase in G expression. Furthermore, it will be of importance to determine to which degree an extended G_{J3666}65U protein initiated at AUG_{29} is produced.

Lastly, whereas this book focused on functional differences in the PVM G gene, structural differences in the M and SH genes were identified. It would be of interest to evaluate these differences in regard to replication efficiency in suitable cells and cell lines, as well as in regard to replication and pathogenicity in vivo. To achieve this, a set of recombinant PVM would be required that in analogy to the G mutants generated for this book that will differ exclusively in the gene of interest. However, this is beyond the scope of this book.

6. References

Ahmadian, G., M. Shamsara, and A.J. Easton. 2005. Pneumoviruses : Molecular Genetics and Reverse Genetics. *Iranian Journal of Biotechnology*. 3:78- 93.

Anderson, L.J., J.C. Hierholzer, C. Tsou, R.M. Hendry, B.F. Fernie, Y. Stone, and K. McIntosh. 1985. Antigenic characterization of respiratory syncytial virus strains with monoclonal antibodies. *J Infect Dis*. 151:626-633.

Anh, D.B., P. Faisca, and D.J. Desmecht. 2006. Differential resistance/susceptibility patterns to pneumovirus infection among inbred mouse strains. *Am J Physiol Lung Cell Mol Physiol*. 291:L426-435.

Arnold, R., B. Konig, H. Werchau, and W. Konig. 2004. Respiratory syncytial virus deficient in soluble G protein induced an increased proinflammatory response in human lung epithelial cells. *Virology*. 330:384-397.

Atreya, P.L., M.E. Peeples, and P.L. Collins. 1998. The NS1 protein of human respiratory syncytial virus is a potent inhibitor of minigenome transcription and RNA replication. *J Virol*. 72:1452-1461.

Banos-Lara Mdel, R., L. Harvey, A. Mendoza, D. Simms, V.N. Chouljenko, N. Wakamatsu, K.G. Kousoulas, and A. Guerrero-Plata. 2015. Impact and regulation of lambda interferon response in human metapneumovirus infection. *J Virol*. 89:730-742.

Bao, X., D. Kolli, J. Ren, T. Liu, R.P. Garofalo, and A. Casola. 2013. Human metapneumovirus glycoprotein G disrupts mitochondrial signaling in airway epithelial cells. *PLoS One*. 8:e62568.

Bao, X., T. Liu, Y. Shan, K. Li, R.P. Garofalo, and A. Casola. 2008. Human metapneumovirus glycoprotein G inhibits innate immune responses. *PLoS Pathog*. 4:e1000077.

Barbosa, C., I. Peixeiro, and L. Romao. 2013. Gene expression regulation by upstream open reading frames and human disease. *PLoS Genet*. 9:e1003529.

Barr, J., P. Chambers, P. Harriott, C.R. Pringle, and A.J. Easton. 1994. Sequence of the phosphoprotein gene of pneumonia virus of mice: expression of multiple proteins from two overlapping reading frames. *J Virol*. 68:5330-5334.

Batonick, M., and G.W. Wertz. 2011. Requirements for Human Respiratory Syncytial Virus Glycoproteins in Assembly and Egress from Infected Cells. *Adv Virol*. 2011.

Becker, S., J. Soukup, and J.R. Yankaskas. 1992. Respiratory syncytial virus infection of human primary nasal and bronchial epithelial cell cultures and bronchoalveolar macrophages. *Am J Respir Cell Mol Biol*. 6:369-374.

Bem, R.A., J.B. Domachowske, and H.F. Rosenberg. 2011. Animal models of human respiratory syncytial virus disease. *Am J Physiol Lung Cell Mol Physiol*. 301:L148-156.

Berthiaume, L., J. Joncas, and V. Pavilanis. 1974. Comparative structure, morphogenesis and biological characteristics of the respiratory syncytial (RS) virus and the pneumonia virus of mice (PVM). *Arch Gesamte Virusforsch*. 45:39-51.

Biacchesi, S., Q.N. Pham, M.H. Skiadopoulos, B.R. Murphy, P.L. Collins, and U.J. Buchholz. 2005. Infection of nonhuman primates with recombinant human metapneumovirus lacking the SH,

G, or M2-2 protein categorizes each as a nonessential accessory protein and identifies vaccine candidates. *J Virol.* 79:12608-12613.

Biacchesi, S., M.H. Skiadopoulos, L. Yang, E.W. Lamirande, K.C. Tran, B.R. Murphy, P.L. Collins, and U.J. Buchholz. 2004. Recombinant human Metapneumovirus lacking the small hydrophobic SH and/or attachment G glycoprotein: deletion of G yields a promising vaccine candidate. *J Virol.* 78:12877-12887.

Bonville, C.A., N.J. Bennett, M. Koehnlein, D.M. Haines, J.A. Ellis, A.M. DelVecchio, H.F. Rosenberg, and J.B. Domachowske. 2006. Respiratory dysfunction and proinflammatory chemokines in the pneumonia virus of mice (PVM) model of viral bronchiolitis. *Virology.* 349:87-95.

Bonville, C.A., N.J. Bennett, C.M. Percopo, P.J. Branigan, A.M. Del Vecchio, H.F. Rosenberg, and J.B. Domachowske. 2007. Diminished inflammatory responses to natural pneumovirus infection among older mice. *Virology.* 368:182-190.

Bourgeois, C., J.B. Bour, K. Lidholt, C. Gauthray, and P. Pothier. 1998. Heparin-like structures on respiratory syncytial virus are involved in its infectivity in vitro. *J Virol.* 72:7221-7227.

Brock, L.G., R.A. Karron, C.D. Krempl, P.L. Collins, and U.J. Buchholz. 2012. Evaluation of pneumonia virus of mice as a possible human pathogen. *J Virol.* 86:5829-5843.

Buchholz, U.J., J.M. Ward, E.W. Lamirande, B. Heinze, C.D. Krempl, and P.L. Collins. 2009. Deletion of nonstructural proteins NS1 and NS2 from pneumonia virus of mice attenuates viral replication and reduces pulmonary cytokine expression and disease. *J Virol.* 83:1969-1980.

Bukreyev, A., S.S. Whitehead, B.R. Murphy, and P.L. Collins. 1997. Recombinant respiratory syncytial virus from which the entire SH gene has been deleted grows efficiently in cell culture and exhibits site-specific attenuation in the respiratory tract of the mouse. *J Virol.* 71:8973-8982.

Bukreyev, A., L. Yang, and P.L. Collins. 2012. The secreted G protein of human respiratory syncytial virus antagonizes antibody-mediated restriction of replication involving macrophages and complement. *J Virol.* 86:10880-10884.

Bukreyev, A., L. Yang, J. Fricke, L. Cheng, J.M. Ward, B.R. Murphy, and P.L. Collins. 2008. The secreted form of respiratory syncytial virus G glycoprotein helps the virus evade antibody-mediated restriction of replication by acting as an antigen decoy and through effects on Fc receptor-bearing leukocytes. *J Virol.* 82:12191-12204.

Calvo, S.E., D.J. Pagliarini, and V.K. Mootha. 2009. Upstream open reading frames cause widespread reduction of protein expression and are polymorphic among humans. *Proc Natl Acad Sci U S A.* 106:7507-7512.

Cartee, T.L., A.G. Megaw, A.G.P. Oomens, and G.W. Wertz. 2003. Identification of a Single Amino Acid Change in the Human Respiratory Syncytial Virus L Protein That Affects Transcriptional Termination. *J Virol.* 77:7352-7360.

Carthew, P., and S. Sparrow. 1980. Persistence of pneumonia virus of mice and Sendai virus in germ-free (nu/nu) mice. *Br J Exp Pathol.* 61:172-175.

Cash, P., C.M. Preston, and C.R. Pringle. 1979. Characterisation of murine pneumonia virus proteins. *Virology.* 96:442-452.

Cash, P., W.H. Wunner, and C.R. Pringle. 1977. A comparison of the polypeptides of human and bovine respiratory syncytial viruses and murine pneumonia virus. *Virology*. 82:369-379.

Cattaneo, R., A. Schmid, D. Eschle, K. Baczko, V. ter Meulen, and M.A. Billeter. 1988. Biased hypermutation and other genetic changes in defective measles viruses in human brain infections. *Cell*. 55:255-265.

Cattaneo, R., A. Schmid, P. Spielhofer, K. Kaelin, K. Baczko, V. ter Meulen, J. Pardowitz, S. Flanagan, B.K. Rima, S.A. Udem, and et al. 1989. Mutated and hypermutated genes of persistent measles viruses which caused lethal human brain diseases. *Virology*. 173:415-425.

Chambers, P., J. Barr, C.R. Pringle, and A.J. Easton. 1990. Molecular cloning of pneumonia virus of mice. *J Virol*. 64:1869-1872.

Chambers, P., D.A. Matthews, C.R. Pringle, and A.J. Easton. 1991. The nucleotide sequences of intergenic regions between nine genes of pneumonia virus of mice establish the physical order of these genes in the viral genome. *Virus Res*. 18:263-270.

Chambers, P., C.R. Pringle, and A.J. Easton. 1992. Sequence analysis of the gene encoding the fusion glycoprotein of pneumonia virus of mice suggests possible conserved secondary structure elements in paramyxovirus fusion glycoproteins. *J Gen Virol*. 73 (Pt 7):1717-1724.

Chauhan, J.S., A. Rao, and G.P. Raghava. 2013. In silico platform for prediction of N-, O- and C-glycosites in eukaryotic protein sequences. *PLoS One*. 8:e67008.

Claassen, E.A., G.M. van Bleek, Z.S. Rychnavska, R.J. de Groot, E.J. Hensen, E.J. Tijhaar, W. van Eden, and R.G. van der Most. 2007. Identification of a CD4 T cell epitope in the pneumonia virus of mice glycoprotein and characterization of its role in protective immunity. *Virology*. 368:17-25.

Collins, P.L. 2011. Human Respiratory Syncytial Virus. *In* The Biology of Paramyxoviruses. S.K. Samal, editor. Caister Academic Press, Norfolk, United Kingdom. 341 - 410.

Collins, P.L., E. Camargo, and M.G. Hill. 1999. Support plasmids and support proteins required for recovery of recombinant respiratory syncytial virus. *Virology*. 259:251-255.

Collins, P.L., and J.E. Crowe. 2006. Respiratory Syncytial Virus and Metapneumovirus. *In* Fields Virology. D. Knipe, P. Howley, D. Griffin, R. Lamb, and M. Malcolm, editors. Lippincott Williams and Wilkins, Philadelphia, PA. 1601- 1646.

Collins, P.L., and B.S. Graham. 2008. Viral and host factors in human respiratory syncytial virus pathogenesis. *J Virol*. 82:2040-2055.

Collins, P.L., M.A. Mink, M.G. Hill, 3rd, E. Camargo, H. Grosfeld, and D.S. Stec. 1993. Rescue of a 7502-nucleotide (49.3% of full-length) synthetic analog of respiratory syncytial virus genomic RNA. *Virology*. 195:252-256.

Collins, P.L., and G. Mottet. 1993. Membrane orientation and oligomerization of the small hydrophobic protein of human respiratory syncytial virus. *J Gen Virol*. 74 (Pt 7):1445-1450.

Compans, R.W., D.H. Harter, and P.W. Choppin. 1967. Studies on pneumonia virus of mice (PVM) in cell culture. II. Structure and morphogenesis of the virus particle. *J Exp Med*. 126:267-276.

Conzelmann, K.-K. 2013. Reverse Genetics of Mononegavirales: The Rabies Virus Paradigm. *In* Sendai Virus Vector. Y. Nagai, editor. Springer Japan. 1-20.

Cook, P.M., R.P. Eglin, and A.J. Easton. 1998. Pathogenesis of pneumovirus infections in mice: detection of pneumonia virus of mice and human respiratory syncytial virus mRNA in lungs of infected mice by in situ hybridization. *J Gen Virol.* 79 (Pt 10):2411-2417.

Curran, J., and D. Kolakofsky. 1999. Replication of paramyxoviruses. *Adv Virus Res.* 54:403-422.

Decaro, N., P. Pinto, V. Mari, G. Elia, V. Larocca, M. Camero, V. Terio, M. Losurdo, V. Martella, and C. Buonavoglia. 2014. Full-genome analysis of a canine pneumovirus causing acute respiratory disease in dogs, Italy. *PLoS One.* 9:e85220.

Dermine, M., and D. Desmecht. 2012. In Vivo modulation of the innate response to pneumovirus by type-I and -III interferon-induced Bos taurus Mx1. *J Interferon Cytokine Res.* 32:332-337.

Derscheid, R.J., and M.R. Ackermann. 2012. Perinatal lamb model of respiratory syncytial virus (RSV) infection. *Viruses.* 4:2359-2378.

Dibben, O., and A.J. Easton. 2007. Mutational analysis of the gene start sequences of pneumonia virus of mice. *Virus Res.* 130:303-309.

Dibben, O., L.C. Thorpe, and A.J. Easton. 2008. Roles of the PVM M2-1, M2-2 and P gene ORF 2 (P-2) proteins in viral replication. *Virus Res.* 131:47-53.

Dickens, L.E., P.L. Collins, and G.W. Wertz. 1984. Transcriptional mapping of human respiratory syncytial virus. *J Virol.* 52:364-369.

Domachowske, J.B., C.A. Bonville, A.J. Easton, and H.F. Rosenberg. 2002. Differential expression of proinflammatory cytokine genes in vivo in response to pathogenic and nonpathogenic pneumovirus infections. *J Infect Dis.* 186:8-14.

Dyer, K., K. Garcia-Crespo, S. Glineur, J. Domachowske, and H. Rosenberg. 2012. The Pneumonia Virus of Mice (PVM) Model of Acute Respiratory Infection. *Viruses.* 4:3494-3510.

Dyer, K.D., R.A. Drummond, T.A. Rice, C.M. Percopo, T.A. Brenner, D.A. Barisas, K.A. Karpe, M.L. Moore, and H.F. Rosenberg. 2015. Priming of the Respiratory Tract with Immunobiotic Lactobacillus plantarum Limits Infection of Alveolar Macrophages with Recombinant Pneumonia Virus of Mice (rK2-PVM). *J Virol.*

Dyer, K.D., I.M. Schellens, C.A. Bonville, B.V. Martin, J.B. Domachowske, and H.F. Rosenberg. 2007. Efficient replication of pneumonia virus of mice (PVM) in a mouse macrophage cell line. *Virol J.* 4:48.

Easton, A.J., and P. Chambers. 1997. Nucleotide sequence of the genes encoding the matrix and small hydrophobic proteins of pneumonia virus of mice. *Virus Res.* 48:27-33.

Easton, A.J., J.B. Domachowske, and H.F. Rosenberg. 2006. Pneumonia Virus of Mice. *In* Perspectives in Medical Virology. Vol. Volume 14. C. Patricia, editor. Elsevier. 299-320.

Edworthy, N.L., and A.J. Easton. 2005. Mutational analysis of the avian pneumovirus conserved transcriptional gene start sequence identifying critical residues. *J Gen Virol.* 86:3343-3347.

Ellis, J.A., B.V. Martin, C. Waldner, K.D. Dyer, J.B. Domachowske, and H.F. Rosenberg. 2007. Mucosal inoculation with an attenuated mouse pneumovirus strain protects against virulent challenge in wild type and interferon-gamma receptor deficient mice. *Vaccine.* 25:1085-1095.

Escribano-Romero, E., J. Rawling, B. Garcia-Barreno, and J.A. Melero. 2004. The Soluble Form of Human Respiratory Syncytial Virus Attachment Protein Differs from the Membrane-Bound

Form in Its Oligomeric State but Is Still Capable of Binding to Cell Surface Proteoglycans. *J Virol.* 78:3524-3532.

Eshaghi, A., V.R. Duvvuri, R. Lai, J.T. Nadarajah, A. Li, S.N. Patel, D.E. Low, and J.B. Gubbay. 2012. Genetic variability of human respiratory syncytial virus A strains circulating in Ontario: a novel genotype with a 72 nucleotide G gene duplication. *PLoS One.* 7:e32807.

Fearns, R., and P.L. Collins. 1999. Role of the M2-1 transcription antitermination protein of respiratory syncytial virus in sequential transcription. *J Virol.* 73:5852-5864.

Fearns, R., P.L. Collins, and M.E. Peeples. 2000. Functional analysis of the genomic and antigenomic promoters of human respiratory syncytial virus. *J Virol.* 74:6006-6014.

Fearns, R., M.E. Peeples, and P.L. Collins. 1997. Increased expression of the N protein of respiratory syncytial virus stimulates minigenome replication but does not alter the balance between the synthesis of mRNA and antigenome. *Virology.* 236:188-201.

Fearns, R., M.E. Peeples, and P.L. Collins. 2002. Mapping the Transcription and Replication Promoters of Respiratory Syncytial Virus. *J Virol.* 76:1663-1672.

Feldman, S.A., R.L. Crim, S.A. Audet, and J.A. Beeler. 2001. Human respiratory syncytial virus surface glycoproteins F, G and SH form an oligomeric complex. *Arch Virol.* 146:2369-2383.

Feldman, S.A., R.M. Hendry, and J.A. Beeler. 1999. Identification of a linear heparin binding domain for human respiratory syncytial virus attachment glycoprotein G. *J Virol.* 73:6610-6617.

Ferreira, J.P., K.W. Overton, and C.L. Wang. 2013. Tuning gene expression with synthetic upstream open reading frames. *Proc Natl Acad Sci U S A.* 110:11284-11289.

Frey, S., C.D. Krempl, A. Schmitt-Graff, and S. Ehl. 2008. Role of T cells in virus control and disease after infection with pneumonia virus of mice. *J Virol.* 82:11619-11627.

Fuentes, S., K.C. Tran, P. Luthra, M.N. Teng, and B. He. 2007. Function of the respiratory syncytial virus small hydrophobic protein. *J Virol.* 81:8361-8366.

Futterer, J., and T. Hohn. 1992. Role of an upstream open reading frame in the translation of polycistronic mRNAs in plant cells. *Nucleic Acids Res.* 20:3851-3857.

Gallaspy, S.E., J.E. Coward, and C. Howe. 1978. Persistent infection of BHK-21 cells with pneumonia virus of mice. *J Virol.* 26:110-114.

Garcia-Barreno, B., C. Palomo, C. Penas, T. Delgado, P. Perez-Brena, and J.A. Melero. 1989. Marked differences in the antigenic structure of human respiratory syncytial virus F and G glycoproteins. *J Virol.* 63:925-932.

Garcia-Beato, R., I. Martinez, C. Franci, F.X. Real, B. Garcia-Barreno, and J.A. Melero. 1996. Host cell effect upon glycosylation and antigenicity of human respiratory syncytial virus G glycoprotein. *Virology.* 221:301-309.

Garcia-Sastre, A., and P. Palese. 1995. The cytoplasmic tail of the neuraminidase protein of influenza A virus does not play an important role in the packaging of this protein into viral envelopes. *Virus Res.* 37:37-47.

Ghildyal, R., C. Baulch-Brown, J. Mills, and J. Meanger. 2003. The matrix protein of Human respiratory syncytial virus localises to the nucleus of infected cells and inhibits transcription. *Arch Virol.* 148:1419-1429.

Ghildyal, R., A. Ho, M. Dias, L. Soegiyono, P.G. Bardin, K.C. Tran, M.N. Teng, and D.A. Jans. 2009. The respiratory syncytial virus matrix protein possesses a Crm1-mediated nuclear export mechanism. *J Virol*. 83:5353-5362.

Ghildyal, R., A. Ho, and D.A. Jans. 2006. Central role of the respiratory syncytial virus matrix protein in infection. *FEMS Microbiol Rev*. 30:692-705.

Ghildyal, R., A. Ho, K.M. Wagstaff, M.M. Dias, C.L. Barton, P. Jans, P. Bardin, and D.A. Jans. 2005a. Nuclear import of the respiratory syncytial virus matrix protein is mediated by importin beta1 independent of importin alpha. *Biochemistry*. 44:12887-12895.

Ghildyal, R., D. Li, I. Peroulis, B. Shields, P.G. Bardin, M.N. Teng, P.L. Collins, J. Meanger, and J. Mills. 2005b. Interaction between the respiratory syncytial virus G glycoprotein cytoplasmic domain and the matrix protein. *J Gen Virol*. 86:1879-1884.

Ghildyal, R., J. Mills, M. Murray, N. Vardaxis, and J. Meanger. 2002. Respiratory syncytial virus matrix protein associates with nucleocapsids in infected cells. *J Gen Virol*. 83:753-757.

Ginsberg, H.S., and F.L. Horsfall, Jr. 1951. Characteristics of the multiplication cycle of pneumonia virus of mice (PVM). *J Exp Med*. 93:151-160.

Glineur, S.F., A.B. Bowen, C.M. Percopo, K.E. Garcia-Crespo, K.D. Dyer, S.I. Ochkur, N.A. Lee, J.J. Lee, J.B. Domachowske, and H.F. Rosenberg. 2014. Sustained inflammation and differential expression of interferons type I and III in PVM-infected interferon-gamma (IFNgamma) gene-deleted mice. *Virology*. 468-470:140-149.

Glineur, S.F., R.W. Renshaw, C.M. Percopo, K.D. Dyer, E.J. Dubovi, J.B. Domachowske, and H.F. Rosenberg. 2013. Novel pneumoviruses (PnVs): Evolution and inflammatory pathology. *Virology*. 443:257-264.

Hallak, L.K., P.L. Collins, W. Knudson, and M.E. Peeples. 2000a. Iduronic acid-containing glycosaminoglycans on target cells are required for efficient respiratory syncytial virus infection. *Virology*. 271:264-275.

Hallak, L.K., D. Spillmann, P.L. Collins, and M.E. Peeples. 2000b. Glycosaminoglycan sulfation requirements for respiratory syncytial virus infection. *J Virol*. 74:10508-10513.

Hardy, R.W., S.B. Harmon, and G.W. Wertz. 1999. Diverse gene junctions of respiratory syncytial virus modulate the efficiency of transcription termination and respond differently to M2-mediated antitermination. *J Virol*. 73:170-176.

Harter, D.H., and P.W. Choppin. 1967. Studies on pneumonia virus of mice (PVM) in cell culture. I. Replication in baby hamster kidney cells and properties of the virus. *J Exp Med*. 126:251-266.

Hartley, J.W., L.H. Evans, K.Y. Green, Z. Naghashfar, A.R. Macias, P.M. Zerfas, and J.M. Ward. 2008. Expression of infectious murine leukemia viruses by RAW264.7 cells, a potential complication for studies with a widely used mouse macrophage cell line. *Retrovirology*. 5:1.

Heinze, B., S. Frey, M. Mordstein, A. Schmitt-Graff, S. Ehl, U.J. Buchholz, P.L. Collins, P. Staeheli, and C.D. Krempl. 2011. Both nonstructural proteins NS1 and NS2 of pneumonia virus of mice are inhibitors of the interferon type I and type III responses in vivo. *J Virol*. 85:4071-4084.

Henderson, G., J. Murray, and R.P. Yeo. 2002. Sorting of the Respiratory Syncytial Virus Matrix Protein into Detergent-Resistant Structures Is Dependent on Cell-Surface Expression of the Glycoproteins. *Virology*. 300:244-254.

Hendricks, D.A., K. Baradaran, K. McIntosh, and J.L. Patterson. 1987. Appearance of a soluble form of the G protein of respiratory syncytial virus in fluids of infected cells. *J Gen Virol*. 68 (Pt 6):1705-1714.

Hendricks, D.A., K. McIntosh, and J.L. Patterson. 1988. Further characterization of the soluble form of the G glycoprotein of respiratory syncytial virus. *J Virol*. 62:2228-2233.

Hofmann, M.A., S.D. Senanayake, and D.A. Brian. 1993. A translation-attenuating intraleader open reading frame is selected on coronavirus mRNAs during persistent infection. *Proc Natl Acad Sci U S A*. 90:11733-11737.

Holder, B.P., P. Simon, L.E. Liao, Y. Abed, X. Bouhy, C.A. Beauchemin, and G. Boivin. 2011. Assessing the in vitro fitness of an oseltamivir-resistant seasonal A/H1N1 influenza strain using a mathematical model. *PLoS One*. 6:e14767.

Hopps, H.E., B.C. Bernheim, A. Nisalak, J.H. Tjio, and J.E. Smadel. 1963. Biologic Characteristics of a Continuous Kidney Cell Line Derived from the African Green Monkey. *J Immunol*. 91:416-424.

Horsfall, F.L., and E.C. Curnen. 1946. Studies on Pneumonia Virus of Mice (Pvm) : Ii. Immunological Evidence of Latent Infection with the Virus in Numerous Mammalian Species. *J Exp Med*. 83:43-64.

Horsfall, F.L., and R.G. Hahn. 1939. A Pneumonia Virus of Swiss Mice. *Experimental Biology and Medicine*. 40:684-686.

Horsfall, F.L., and R.G. Hahn. 1940. A Latent Virus in Normal Mice Capable of Producing Pneumonia in Its Natural Host. *J Exp Med*. 71:391-408.

Horsfall, F.L., Jr., and H.S. Ginsberg. 1951. The dependence of the pathological lesion upon the multiplication of pneumonia virus of mice (PVM); kinetic relation between the degree of viral multiplication and the extent of pneumonia. *J Exp Med*. 93:139-150.

Johnson, P.R., M.K. Spriggs, R.A. Olmsted, and P.L. Collins. 1987. The G glycoprotein of human respiratory syncytial viruses of subgroups A and B: extensive sequence divergence between antigenically related proteins. *Proc Natl Acad Sci U S A*. 84:5625-5629.

Johnson, T.R., J.E. Johnson, S.R. Roberts, G.W. Wertz, R.A. Parker, and B.S. Graham. 1998. Priming with secreted glycoprotein G of respiratory syncytial virus (RSV) augments interleukin-5 production and tissue eosinophilia after RSV challenge. *J Virol*. 72:2871-2880.

Karger, A., U. Schmidt, and U.J. Buchholz. 2001. Recombinant bovine respiratory syncytial virus with deletions of the G or SH genes: G and F proteins bind heparin. *J Gen Virol*. 82:631-640.

Karron, R.A., P.F. Wright, J.E. Crowe, Jr., M.L. Clements-Mann, J. Thompson, M. Makhene, R. Casey, and B.R. Murphy. 1997. Evaluation of two live, cold-passaged, temperature-sensitive respiratory syncytial virus vaccines in chimpanzees and in human adults, infants, and children. *J Infect Dis*. 176:1428-1436.

King, A.M., E. Lefkowitz, M.J. Adams, and E.B. Carstens. 2012. Virus Taxonomy: Classification and Nomenclature of Viruses. Ninth Report of the International Committee on Taxonomy of Viruses. Elsevier Academic Press, San Diego, CA.

Kozak, M. 1987. An analysis of 5'-noncoding sequences from 699 vertebrate messenger RNAs. *Nucleic Acids Res*. 15:8125-8148.

Kozak, M. 1999. Initiation of translation in prokaryotes and eukaryotes. *Gene*. 234:187-208.

Kozak, M. 2002. Pushing the limits of the scanning mechanism for initiation of translation. *Gene*. 299:1-34.

Kozak, M. 2005. Regulation of translation via mRNA structure in prokaryotes and eukaryotes. *Gene*. 361:13-37.

Krempl, C.D., and P.L. Collins. 2004. Reevaluation of the virulence of prototypic strain 15 of pneumonia virus of mice. *J Virol*. 78:13362-13365.

Krempl, C.D., E.W. Lamirande, and P.L. Collins. 2005. Complete sequence of the RNA genome of pneumonia virus of mice (PVM). *Virus Genes*. 30:237-249.

Krempl, C.D., A. Wnekowicz, E.W. Lamirande, G. Nayebagha, P.L. Collins, and U.J. Buchholz. 2007. Identification of a novel virulence factor in recombinant pneumonia virus of mice. *J Virol*. 81:9490-9501.

Krusat, T., and H.J. Streckert. 1997. Heparin-dependent attachment of respiratory syncytial virus (RSV) to host cells. *Arch Virol*. 142:1247-1254.

Kuo, L., R. Fearns, and P.L. Collins. 1996a. The structurally diverse intergenic regions of respiratory syncytial virus do not modulate sequential transcription by a dicistronic minigenome. *J Virol*. 70:6143-6150.

Kuo, L., R. Fearns, and P.L. Collins. 1997. Analysis of the gene start and gene end signals of human respiratory syncytial virus: quasi-templated initiation at position 1 of the encoded mRNA. *J Virol*. 71:4944-4953.

Kuo, L., H. Grosfeld, J. Cristina, M.G. Hill, and P.L. Collins. 1996b. Effects of mutations in the gene-start and gene-end sequence motifs on transcription of monocistronic and dicistronic minigenomes of respiratory syncytial virus. *J Virol*. 70:6892-6901.

Kwilas, S., R.M. Liesman, L. Zhang, E. Walsh, R.J. Pickles, and M.E. Peeples. 2009. Respiratory syncytial virus grown in Vero cells contains a truncated attachment protein that alters its infectivity and dependence on glycosaminoglycans. *J Virol*. 83:10710-10718.

Laemmli, U.K. 1970. Cleavage of Structural Proteins during the Assembly of the Head of Bacteriophage T4. *Nature*. 227:680-685.

Lambert, D.M. 1988. Role of oligosaccharides in the structure and function of respiratory syncytial virus glycoproteins. *Virology*. 164:458-466.

Latiff, K., J. Meanger, J. Mills, and R. Ghildyal. 2004. Sequence and structure relatedness of matrix protein of human respiratory syncytial virus with matrix proteins of other negative-sense RNA viruses. *Clin Microbiol Infect*. 10:945-948.

Le Nouen, C., P. Hillyer, L.G. Brock, C.C. Winter, R.L. Rabin, P.L. Collins, and U.J. Buchholz. 2014. Human metapneumovirus SH and G glycoproteins inhibit macropinocytosis-mediated entry into human dendritic cells and reduce CD4+ T cell activation. *J Virol*. 88:6453-6469.

Levine, S., R. Klaiber-Franco, and P.R. Paradiso. 1987. Demonstration that glycoprotein G is the attachment protein of respiratory syncytial virus. *J Gen Virol*. 68 (Pt 9):2521-2524.

Li, D., D.A. Jans, P.G. Bardin, J. Meanger, J. Mills, and R. Ghildyal. 2008. Association of respiratory syncytial virus M protein with viral nucleocapsids is mediated by the M2-1 protein. *J Virol*. 82:8863-8870.

Ling, R., and C.R. Pringle. 1989a. Polypeptides of pneumonia virus of mice. I. Immunological cross-reactions and post-translational modifications. *J Gen Virol*. 70 (Pt 6):1427-1440.

Ling, R., and C.R. Pringle. 1989b. Polypeptides of pneumonia virus of mice. II. Characterization of the glycoproteins. *J Gen Virol*. 70 (Pt 6):1441-1452.

Ling, R., S. Sinkovic, D. Toquin, O. Guionie, N. Eterradossi, and A.J. Easton. 2008. Deletion of the SH gene from avian metapneumovirus has a greater impact on virus production and immunogenicity in turkeys than deletion of the G gene or M2-2 open reading frame. *J Gen Virol*. 89:525-533.

Low, K.W., T. Tan, K. Ng, B.H. Tan, and R.J. Sugrue. 2008. The RSV F and G glycoproteins interact to form a complex on the surface of infected cells. *Biochem Biophys Res Commun*. 366:308-313.

Madarame, H., K. Ogihara, M. Kimura, M. Nagai, T. Omatsu, H. Ochiai, and T. Mizutani. 2014. Detection of a pneumonia virus of mice (PVM) in an African hedgehog (Atelerix arbiventris) with suspected wobbly hedgehog syndrome (WHS). *Vet Microbiol*. 173:136-140.

Maher, C.F., T. Hussell, E. Blair, C.J. Ring, and P.J. Openshaw. 2004. Recombinant respiratory syncytial virus lacking secreted glycoprotein G is attenuated, non-pathogenic but induces protective immunity. *Microbes Infect*. 6:1049-1055.

Marino, J.H., P. Cook, and K.S. Miller. 2003. Accurate and statistically verified quantification of relative mRNA abundances using SYBR Green I and real-time RT-PCR. *Journal of Immunological Methods*. 283:291-306.

Marty, A., J. Meanger, J. Mills, B. Shields, and R. Ghildyal. 2004. Association of matrix protein of respiratory syncytial virus with the host cell membrane of infected cells. *Arch Virol*. 149:199-210.

McLellan, J.S., W.C. Ray, and M.E. Peeples. 2013. Structure and function of respiratory syncytial virus surface glycoproteins. *Curr Top Microbiol Immunol*. 372:83-104.

Meijer, H.A., and A.A. Thomas. 2002. Control of eukaryotic protein synthesis by upstream open reading frames in the 5'-untranslated region of an mRNA. *Biochem J*. 367:1-11.

Melendi, G.A., D. Bridget, A.C. Monsalvo, F.F. Laham, P. Acosta, M.F. Delgado, F.P. Polack, and P.M. Irusta. 2011. Conserved cysteine residues within the attachment G glycoprotein of respiratory syncytial virus play a critical role in the enhancement of cytotoxic T-lymphocyte responses. *Virus Genes*. 42:46-54.

Melero, J.A., B. Garcia-Barreno, I. Martinez, C.R. Pringle, and P.A. Cane. 1997. Antigenic structure, evolution and immunobiology of human respiratory syncytial virus attachment (G) protein. *J Gen Virol*. 78 (Pt 10):2411-2418.

Mitchell, J.A., J.M. Cardwell, R.W. Renshaw, E.J. Dubovi, and J. Brownlie. 2013. Detection of canine pneumovirus in dogs with canine infectious respiratory disease. *J Clin Microbiol*. 51:4112-4119.

Mitnaul, L.J., M.R. Castrucci, K.G. Murti, and Y. Kawaoka. 1996. The cytoplasmic tail of influenza A virus neuraminidase (NA) affects NA incorporation into virions, virion morphology, and virulence in mice but is not essential for virus replication. *J Virol*. 70:873-879.

Mitra, R., P. Baviskar, R.R. Duncan-Decocq, D. Patel, and A.G. Oomens. 2012. The human respiratory syncytial virus matrix protein is required for maturation of viral filaments. *J Virol.* 86:4432-4443.

Miyata, H., M. Kishikawa, H. Kondo, C. Kai, Y. Watanabe, K. Ohsawa, and H. Sato. 1995. New isolates of pneumonia virus of mice (PVM) from Japanese rat colonies and their characterization. *Exp Anim.* 44:95-104.

Miyata, H., Y. Watanabe, H. Kondo, K. Yagami, and H. Sato. 1993. Serological evidence of pneumonia virus of mouse (PVM) infection in laboratory rats. *Jikken Dobutsu.* 42:371-376.

Moudy, R.M., S.B. Harmon, W.M. Sullender, and G.W. Wertz. 2003. Variations in transcription termination signals of human respiratory syncytial virus clinical isolates affect gene expression. *Virology.* 313:250-260.

Moudy, R.M., W.M. Sullender, and G.W. Wertz. 2004. Variations in intergenic region sequences of Human respiratory syncytial virus clinical isolates: analysis of effects on transcriptional regulation. *Virology.* 327:121-133.

Mufson, M.A., C. Orvell, B. Rafnar, and E. Norrby. 1985. Two distinct subtypes of human respiratory syncytial virus. *J Gen Virol.* 66 (Pt 10):2111-2124.

Peeples, M.E., and P.L. Collins. 2000. Mutations in the 5' trailer region of a respiratory syncytial virus minigenome which limit RNA replication to one step. *J Virol.* 74:146-155.

Percopo, C.M., E.J. Dubovi, R.W. Renshaw, K.D. Dyer, J.B. Domachowske, and H.F. Rosenberg. 2011. Canine pneumovirus replicates in mouse lung tissue and elicits inflammatory pathology. *Virology.* 416:26-31.

Pringle, C.R., and R.P. Eglin. 1986. Murine pneumonia virus: seroepidemiological evidence of widespread human infection. *J Gen Virol.* 67 (Pt 6):975-982.

Pringle, C.R., and J.E. Parry. 1980. Location and quantitation of antigen on the surface of virusinfected cells by specific bacterial adherence and scanning electron microscopy. *J Virol Methods.* 1:61-75.

Randhawa, J.S., P. Chambers, C.R. Pringle, and A.J. Easton. 1995. Nucleotide sequences of the genes encoding the putative attachment glycoprotein (G) of mouse and tissue culture-passaged strains of pneumonia virus of mice. *Virology.* 207:240-245.

Renshaw, R., M. Laverack, N. Zylich, A. Glaser, and E. Dubovi. 2011. Genomic analysis of a pneumovirus isolated from dogs with acute respiratory disease. *Vet Microbiol.* 150:88-95.

Renshaw, R.W., N.C. Zylich, M.A. Laverack, A.L. Glaser, and E.J. Dubovi. 2010. Pneumovirus in dogs with acute respiratory disease. *Emerg Infect Dis.* 16:993-995.

Richter, C.B., J.E. Thigpen, C.S. Richter, and J.M. Mackenzie, Jr. 1988. Fatal pneumonia with terminal emaciation in nude mice caused by pneumonia virus of mice. *Lab Anim Sci.* 38:255-261.

Rosenberg, H.F., C.A. Bonville, A.J. Easton, and J.B. Domachowske. 2005. The pneumonia virus of mice infection model for severe respiratory syncytial virus infection: identifying novel targets for therapeutic intervention. *Pharmacol Ther.* 105:1-6.

Rosenberg, H.F., and J.B. Domachowske. 2008. Pneumonia virus of mice: severe respiratory infection in a natural host. *Immunol Lett.* 118:6-12.

Rueda, P., B. Garcia-Barreno, and J.A. Melero. 1994. Loss of conserved cysteine residues in the attachment (G) glycoprotein of two human respiratory syncytial virus escape mutants that contain multiple A-G substitutions (hypermutations). *Virology*. 198:653-662.

Ruijter, J.M., C. Ramakers, W.M. Hoogaars, Y. Karlen, O. Bakker, M.J. van den Hoff, and A.F. Moorman. 2009. Amplification efficiency: linking baseline and bias in the analysis of quantitative PCR data. *Nucleic Acids Res*. 37:e45.

Schiff, L.J. 1976. Replication of murine paramyxoviruses in hamster tracheal organ culture and comparison with standard tissue culture methods. *J Clin Microbiol*. 4:248-252.

Schlender, J., G. Zimmer, G. Herrler, and K.K. Conzelmann. 2003. Respiratory Syncytial Virus (RSV) Fusion Protein Subunit F2, Not Attachment Protein G, Determines the Specificity of RSV Infection. *J Virol*. 77:4609-4616.

Schmidt, U., J. Beyer, U. Polster, L.J. Gershwin, and U.J. Buchholz. 2002. Mucosal Immunization with Live Recombinant Bovine Respiratory Syncytial Virus (BRSV) and Recombinant BRSV Lacking the Envelope Glycoprotein G Protects against Challenge with Wild-Type BRSV. *J Virol*. 76:12355-12359.

Schmitt, A.P., B. He, and R.A. Lamb. 1999. Involvement of the cytoplasmic domain of the hemagglutinin-neuraminidase protein in assembly of the paramyxovirus simian virus 5. *J Virol*. 73:8703-8712.

Schwarze, J. 2004. Enhanced virulence, airway inflammation and impaired lung function induced by respiratory syncytial virus deficient in secreted G protein. *Thorax*. 59:517-521.

Shaikh, F.Y., R.G. Cox, A.W. Lifland, A.L. Hotard, J.V. Williams, M.L. Moore, P.J. Santangelo, and J.E. Crowe, Jr. 2012. A critical phenylalanine residue in the respiratory syncytial virus fusion protein cytoplasmic tail mediates assembly of internal viral proteins into viral filaments and particles. *MBio*. 3.

Shimonaski, G., and P.E. Came. 1970. Plaque assay for pneumonia virus of mice. *Appl Microbiol*. 20:775-777.

Spriggs, M.K., and P.L. Collins. 1990. Intracellular processing and transport of NH2-terminally truncated forms of a hemagglutinin-neuraminidase type II glycoprotein. *J Cell Biol*. 111:31-44.

Stobart, C.C., and M.L. Moore. 2014. RNA virus reverse genetics and vaccine design. *Viruses*. 6:2531-2550.

Taniguchi, K., and S. Komoto. 2012. Genetics and reverse genetics of rotavirus. *Curr Opin Virol*. 2:399-407.

Techaarpornkul, S., N. Barretto, and M.E. Peeples. 2001. Functional analysis of recombinant respiratory syncytial virus deletion mutants lacking the small hydrophobic and/or attachment glycoprotein gene. *J Virol*. 75:6825-6834.

Techaarpornkul, S., P.L. Collins, and M.E. Peeples. 2002. Respiratory syncytial virus with the fusion protein as its only viral glycoprotein is less dependent on cellular glycosaminoglycans for attachment than complete virus. *Virology*. 294:296-304.

Teng, M.N., and P.L. Collins. 1998. Identification of the respiratory syncytial virus proteins required for formation and passage of helper-dependent infectious particles. *J Virol*. 72:5707-5716.

Teng, M.N., S.S. Whitehead, and P.L. Collins. 2001. Contribution of the respiratory syncytial virus G glycoprotein and its secreted and membrane-bound forms to virus replication in vitro and in vivo. *Virology*. 289:283-296.

Tennant, R.W., and T.G. Ward. 1962. Pneumonia virus of mice (PVM) in cell culture. *Proc Soc Exp Biol Med*. 111:395-398.

Thorpe, L.C., and A.J. Easton. 2005. Genome sequence of the non-pathogenic strain 15 of pneumonia virus of mice and comparison with the genome of the pathogenic strain J3666. *J Gen Virol*. 86:159-169.

Tran, K.C., P.L. Collins, and M.N. Teng. 2004. Effects of altering the transcription termination signals of respiratory syncytial virus on viral gene expression and growth in vitro and in vivo. *J Virol*. 78:692-699.

Trento, A., M. Galiano, C. Videla, G. Carballal, B. Garcia-Barreno, J.A. Melero, and C. Palomo. 2003. Major changes in the G protein of human respiratory syncytial virus isolates introduced by a duplication of 60 nucleotides. *J Gen Virol*. 84:3115-3120.

Triantafilou, K., S. Kar, E. Vakakis, S. Kotecha, and M. Triantafilou. 2013. Human respiratory syncytial virus viroporin SH: a viral recognition pathway used by the host to signal inflammasome activation. *Thorax*. 68:66-75.

Walsh, E.E. 2011. Respiratory syncytial virus infection in adults. *Semin Respir Crit Care Med*. 32:423-432.

Walsh, E.E., A.R. Falsey, and W.M. Sullender. 1998. Monoclonal antibody neutralization escape mutants of respiratory syncytial virus with unique alterations in the attachment (G) protein. *J Gen Virol*. 79 (Pt 3):479-487.

Walsh, K.B., J. Sidney, M. Welch, D.M. Fremgen, A. Sette, and M.B. Oldstone. 2013. CD8+ T-cell epitope mapping for pneumonia virus of mice in H-2b mice. *J Virol*. 87:9949-9952.

Waris, M. 1991. Pattern of respiratory syncytial virus epidemics in Finland: two-year cycles with alternating prevalence of groups A and B. *J Infect Dis*. 163:464-469.

Watkiss, E.R., P. Shrivastava, N. Arsic, S. Gomis, and S. van Drunen Littel-van den Hurk. 2013. Innate and adaptive immune response to pneumonia virus of mice in a resistant and a susceptible mouse strain. *Viruses*. 5:295-320.

Weir, E.C., D.G. Brownstein, A.L. Smith, and E.A. Johnson. 1988. Respiratory disease and wasting in athymic mice infected with pneumonia virus of mice. *Lab Anim Sci*. 38:133-137.

Weischenfeldt, J., and B. Porse. 2008. Bone Marrow-Derived Macrophages (BMM): Isolation and Applications. *CSH Protoc*. 2008:pdb prot5080.

Wertz, G.W., P.L. Collins, Y. Huang, C. Gruber, S. Levine, and L.A. Ball. 1985. Nucleotide sequence of the G protein gene of human respiratory syncytial virus reveals an unusual type of viral membrane protein. *Proc Natl Acad Sci U S A*. 82:4075-4079.

Whitehead, S.S., A. Bukreyev, M.N. Teng, C.Y. Firestone, M. St Claire, W.R. Elkins, P.L. Collins, and B.R. Murphy. 1999. Recombinant respiratory syncytial virus bearing a deletion of either the NS2 or SH gene is attenuated in chimpanzees. *J Virol*. 73:3438-3442.

Widjojoatmodjo, M.N., J. Boes, M. van Bers, Y. van Remmerden, P.J. Roholl, and W. Luytjes. 2010. A highly attenuated recombinant human respiratory syncytial virus lacking the G protein induces long-lasting protection in cotton rats. *Virol J.* 7:114.

Wilson, C., R. Gilmore, and T. Morrison. 1990. Aberrant membrane insertion of a cytoplasmic tail deletion mutant of the hemagglutinin-neuraminidase glycoprotein of Newcastle disease virus. *Molecular and Cellular Biology.* 10:449-457.

Wong, T.C., M. Ayata, S. Ueda, and A. Hirano. 1991. Role of biased hypermutation in evolution of subacute sclerosing panencephalitis virus from progenitor acute measles virus. *J Virol.* 65:2191-2199.

Zenner, L., and J.P. Regnault. 2000. Ten-year long monitoring of laboratory mouse and rat colonies in French facilities: a retrospective study. *Laboratory Animals.* 34:76-83.

Zhang, J., G.P. Leser, A. Pekosz, and R.A. Lamb. 2000. The cytoplasmic tails of the influenza virus spike glycoproteins are required for normal genome packaging. *Virology.* 269:325-334.

www.ingramcontent.com/pod-product-compliance
Lightning Source LLC
LaVergne TN
LVHW091038150826
845672LV00006BA/1873

* 9 7 8 3 3 8 4 2 6 5 0 6 7 *